WHAT PATIENTS SAY,
WHAT DOCTORS HEAR

For Naava, Noah,
and Ariel

WHAT PATIENTS SAY, WHAT DOCTORS HEAR

Danielle Ofri, MD

BEACON PRESS
BOSTON

BEACON PRESS
Boston, Massachusetts
www.beacon.org

Beacon Press books
are published under the auspices of
the Unitarian Universalist Association of Congregations.

19 18 17 16   8 7 6 5 4 3 2 1

This book is printed on acid-free paper that meets the uncoated paper
ANSI/NISO specifications for permanence as revised in 1992.

Text design and composition by Kim Arney

The names of the patients in this book have been changed to protect their identities,
with the exceptions of Morgan Amanda Fritzlen and Tracey Pratt, who consented
to have their real names used. All other names are real.

A few minor parts of this book have appeared in different form
in the *New York Times* and *Los Angeles Times*.

Library of Congress Cataloging-in-Publication Data

Names: Ofri, Danielle, author.
Title: What patients say, what doctors hear / Danielle Ofri.
Description: Boston, Massachusetts : Beacon Press, [2017] |
Includes bibliographical references and index.
Identifiers: LCCN 2016021634 (print) | LCCN 2016022893 (ebook) |
ISBN 9780807062630 (hardcover : alk. paper) | ISBN 9780807062647 (ebook)
Subjects: | MESH: Physician-Patient Relations | Communication
Classification: LCC R727.3 (print) | LCC R727.3 (ebook) | NLM W 62 |
DDC 610.69/6—dc23
LC record available at https://lccn.loc.gov/2016021634

Contents

CHAPTER I

Communication and Its Discontents

It was late on a Thursday evening and I already had one foot out of the clinic door when my office phone rang. It was Oumar Amadou.[1] "I am not feeling well," he said. "I need to see you, Dr. Ofri."

The sun had set and the clinic was closing up. I had already locked up my file cabinets and turned off the computer. "I need to see you now," Mr. Amadou said. The annoyance in his voice was apparent even with his thick West African accent.

In the few months I'd known Mr. Amadou, I'd probably fielded fifty phone calls from him. He always had something bothering him, or needed a form filled out, or a medication refilled, and he always needed it right away. He constantly showed up at the clinic without an appointment, assuming I would be available to see him right then and there.

But he also had a severe heart condition, even though he was only forty-three years old. At our first visit he'd hauled out a tome of papers from a cardiologist in Pittsburgh. The papers detailed a severely malfunctioning heart, one that had required a pacemaker, a defibrillator, and several stays in the ICU.

So when he called on a Thursday evening, I took his concerns seriously, despite the irritating tone of his voice and my depleted reserve of patience for him. I questioned him about his symptoms to see if he might be experiencing congestive heart failure or an arrhythmia—things for which I would send him to the emergency room immediately.

But he had no specific symptoms, just a vague sense of not feeling well. I wasn't scheduled to be in the clinic the following day, Friday, but because of his poor heart I didn't feel comfortable having him wait until Monday.

"Please come to the clinic tomorrow," I said, "to the urgent-care section." I explained that I wouldn't be there but that he would be evaluated by one of my colleagues.

When I arrived on Monday morning there was an indignant voice-mail message from Mr. Amadou. "I come Friday, but you no there, so I go home. I need to see *you*!" My hands slapped into my lap with frustration. Either he hadn't understood what I'd said or he was simply being stubborn.

The next three days were a series of missed phone messages between us. If he was feeling sick, I told him, he should come to urgent care right away. If he didn't feel too bad, we could give him a regular appointment. He left repeated voice mails saying, "I need to see you, Dr. Ofri," seeming not to acknowledge any of my messages to him. Whenever I called back, I got only his voice mail.

Midday on Thursday, just as I was saying good-bye to the last of my morning patients, contemplating the possibility that I might actually have five minutes for lunch, Mr. Amadou popped into my line of sight. It had been a week now that we'd been trading messages. Tall and lanky, dressed in a powder-blue tracksuit, he signaled anxiously at me. "I need to see you, Dr. Ofri," he called out. "It is very important."

I was unprepared for the rush of anger that flooded over me. It wasn't just that I was about to lose that rare opportunity to eat lunch after an exhausting morning, but that Mr. Amadou would just walk in the door and assume I would drop everything and give him a medical evaluation that instant.

Yes, he had a bad heart and all, but that didn't give him a free pass to be so demanding. Obviously, whatever was bothering him couldn't be so bad given that he'd chosen to spend the week trading messages with me rather than come to the urgent-care clinic. I needed to draw a line.

"Mr. Amadou," I said tautly, "you cannot just show up to the clinic without an appointment."

"I come here to see you, Dr. Ofri," he said.

"Yes, I know," I said, growing more exasperated. "But I have other patients with scheduled appointments. If it's something that can't wait, you can use the urgent-care clinic today. Otherwise, you need to make an appointment like everyone else."

"I no see other doctor," Mr. Amadou said. "I only want to see you. I need to see you today."

I knew that if I gave Mr. Amadou a medical visit right now, I'd reinforce the idea that he could simply walk into my office at any time. He'd be at my doorstep every week! But I also understood the severity of his cardiomyopathy—this was not the type of patient I could take a chance on, annoying or not.

"Okay, Mr. Amadou," I said, sighing heavily, "just a quick visit. Next time you must have an appointment."

Mr. Amadou smiled broadly as I led him from the waiting room and I knew I was going to regret this decision. He had now figured out how to get an instant appointment: just be annoyingly persistent until I caved.

The medical assistant was about to leave for lunch also but I gave him a beseeching smile. "Could you please do a quick set of vital signs for Mr. Amadou?" I asked. He hesitated, raised an eyebrow, then finally assented. With relief, I gestured for Mr. Amadou to enter the assistant's room.

Mr. Amadou took two steps and then paused in mid-footfall. It was like a movie that abruptly froze, catching a character in the midst of an action. He seemed to hold his lanky body aloft, almost as though the muscles were debating whether to move it forward or backward. But it was all an illusion, as he collapsed to the floor with a heart-stopping thud.

There is always that dreadful moment of silence—probably less than a second, but it feels like an hour—when you realize something terrible has occurred. It's that stomach-lurching moment as your body and mind are shocked from the ordinary to the emergency. It's a vexing if brief time lag in which you need to blink several times, it seems, before you can accept the new reality.

I dropped to my knees and pressed my fingers to his neck to check a pulse. "Mr. Amadou," I shouted. "Can you hear me?" He was breathing rapidly, his upper back slumped against the door frame, the rest of his lengthy body stretched out in the hallway. "Tell me what's going on. Are you having any pain?" He placed his right hand over his chest. "My heart," he said faintly, and I was swamped with a horrific wave of guilt.

By now a crowd had gathered around. The nurse was checking Mr. Amadou's blood pressure. His pulse was 130. His fingers were so cold that the oxygen saturation monitor could not pick up a reading. I called for oxygen and a stretcher while I crammed my stethoscope under the jacket of his tracksuit. We loaded his listless body onto the stretcher and began wheeling him rapidly to the emergency room.

Disconsolate, I held Mr. Amadou's hand as we pressed down the hall, striding briskly to keep my pangs of remorse at bay, praying that he was going to be okay. We rolled him into the triage bay of the emergency room and I explained the situation to the ER doctor while the nurses hooked up monitors and started an IV. As we finished the handoff of medical care, I turned back again to Mr. Amadou. I took his cool, clammy right hand in my two hands and gave it a squeeze. His fingers were frigid.

I apologized for berating him in the waiting room and for all of our miscommunications during the week. He opened his eyes to my words but was too breathless to speak. He nodded slightly and then squeezed my hand weakly.

I trudged back to the clinic, staring down at the linoleum floor the whole way. Despite my efforts not to, I couldn't hold back from dissecting in minute detail the events that had just transpired, trying to figure out the mistakes. Mr. Amadou had been demanding, probably unreasonably so. And I had put my foot down, perhaps a bit too decisively.

But maybe the problem was more basic than that. Maybe we just weren't hearing each other. True, we had a language barrier, but he navigated fairly well in English, and I used a French interpreter whenever we discussed anything complicated. I didn't really think it was a problem in understanding the actual words, more a problem of hearing what the other person was trying to convey.

For all of his annoying mannerisms and pushiness, Mr. Amadou was fundamentally trying to say, "Help me." Deep down, no doubt, he was terrified that his heart could give out at any moment. This fear informed all of his actions. Seen in this light, his relentlessness was understandable—his life hung in the balance—so he could never take no for an answer.

But his relentlessness was smothering to me. Every time I turned around, it seemed, there was Mr. Amadou jockeying for my time and attention. I wanted to help him but his insistence on being front and center depleted me. I accept that my job requires me to put my patients' needs before my own, but Mr. Amadou's unending demands made me defensive and eventually angry. I could no longer hear what he was saying because I was busy reacting to his forceful behavior. I was expending so much effort drawing a protective line in the sand that I could not hear his pleas for help. I could not make the connection that the very annoyance of his behavior was itself a plea for help, a declaration of fear and vulnerability.

For all of the sophisticated diagnostic tools of modern medicine, the conversation between doctor and patient remains the primary diagnostic tool. Even in the fields that are visually based, such as dermatology, or procedurally based, such as surgery, the patient's verbal description of the problem and the doctor's questions about it are critical to an accurate diagnosis.

In some ways this seems almost anachronistic, given how advanced so much of our technology is now. Science-fiction movies predicted that medical diagnosis would be achieved by running a handheld machine over the patient's body. And indeed much diagnosis is made with MRIs, PET scans, and advanced CT technology. Yet the simple verbal exchange between patient and doctor remains the cornerstone of medical diagnosis. The story the patient tells the doctor constitutes the primary data that guide diagnosis, clinical decision-making, and treatment.

However, the story the patient tells and the story the doctor hears are often not the same thing. The story Mr. Amadou was telling me and the story I was hearing were not identical. There were so many layers of emotion, frustration, logistics, and desperation, that it was almost as if we were in two different conversations entirely.

It is a common complaint of patients. They feel their doctors don't really listen, don't hear what they are trying to say. Many patients leave their medical encounters disappointed and frustrated. But beyond being merely dissatisfied, many patients leave misdiagnosed or improperly treated.

Doctors are equally frustrated with the difficulties of piecing together a patient's story, especially for those with complex and inscrutable symptoms. As medicine grows more complicated, with illnesses more multifold and complex, the gap between what patients say and what doctors hear—and vice versa—grows more significant. I began writing this book to examine these interactions between patients and doctors, to explore how a story traverses from one party to the other.

It's clear that doctors and patients don't start out on equal footing—the patient is the one with the fever, or who is short of breath, or who is panicked that a lump on the neck is cancer. The patient starts out in a more vulnerable position. But, also, the stakes are much higher for the patient, who has far more to lose if things go wrong. So it's fair to say that the doctor bears more of the responsibility in ensuring that the story is understood correctly. Nevertheless, it is still a two-person encounter, with each person bringing his or her own biases, history, strengths, and liabilities.

In Mr. Amadou's case, there were mutual missteps that served to worsen his medical condition. If either or both of us had been better able to listen to the other, perhaps Mr. Amadou might not have ended up in the intensive-care unit that afternoon. Medical care is a shared endeavor and communication is its sine qua non.

In this book I trace the paths of several patients and doctors, examining how a story travels from one human being to another. By exploring the challenges and pitfalls, as well as the collaborations and the successes, I hope to illuminate the role of this most potent diagnostic—and therapeutic—tool in medicine. The more technologically advanced medicine becomes, the more we are reminded of the crucial role of the story.

After Mr. Amadou was safely in the emergency room, I returned to the clinic and saw that the afternoon session was already in full swing. Lunch was long since out of the question, but I'd lost my appetite anyway. Besides, charts were already stacked in my box. The clerk handed me the first one. "Mrs. Velasquez doesn't have an appointment for today but asked if you could squeeze her in."

The impress of Mr. Amadou's chilled hands still seemed to linger in mine. His pleas for help, however frustrating, still echoed in my head. "Whoever shows up," I said, "just add 'em on to the schedule." I took the chart from her hand and geared up for a long afternoon.

Mr. Amadou spent several days in the ICU—a rapid pulse had overwhelmed the ability of his weakened heart muscle to pump effectively. His pacemaker had to be replaced and his medications titrated to a new, fragile equilibrium. He survived this hospitalization but his limited cardiac reserve keeps me in a constant state of worry. Since that day, every time he calls I listen twice as hard. I can feel myself "squinting" my ear into the phone as I try to figure out whether there is something serious underfoot. When we see each other in person at his appointments, our conversation feels almost as corporeal as our physical exam. There is nothing passive or mundane any longer in our communication.

Mr. Amadou serves as my continual reminder that how doctors and patients communicate with one another is not just a pleasantry of good bedside manner but in fact the most critical element of medical care. It can sometimes mean life or death.

CHAPTER 2

From Both Sides Now

Morgan Amanda Fritzlen was a college student in her midtwenties. Juliet Mavromatis was an internist in her midforties. Their paths crossed at the leafy campus of Emory University, where Juliet was an attending physician and Morgan Amanda, a linguistics and health communications undergraduate. Morgan Amanda readily acknowledged she was a "challenging patient," and Juliet would not have disagreed.

Morgan Amanda's childhood had been plagued by all sorts of odd illnesses and injuries. At various times her hands and feet ached, then her ankles and knees, then her shoulders and her neck. The pediatricians reassured her parents that these were growing pains, or caused by a viral syndrome, or remnants of a childhood injury. But injuries occurred with everyday activities. Headaches, dizziness, and lethargy were constant companions and it was difficult for Morgan Amanda to keep up with other kids at the schoolyard. It felt like she was struggling to swim against the stream of life, though her smiling exterior kept this reality private.

She was blessed with long, delicate arms and legs that made her perfect for ballet, but those same lanky limbs seemed to preternaturally twist and trip, causing multiple dislocations. "I'm probably the only person who's ever fractured her arm falling *up* the stairs," Morgan Amanda told me, with a laugh. She managed to twist her ankles while walking on ordinary flat ground. "I was all arms and legs," she said, "graceful but clumsy and accident-prone, if you can imagine such a combination. When I was born my father said I resembled a string chicken!"

Aches and pains occurred in strange locations. Her scalp hurt, for example, whenever her mother brushed her hair. Home movies showed her tugging at her tight bun during ballet recitals. Visual problems necessitated more than a dozen surgeries on her eye muscles. She seemed to catch every bug that went around, be it viral, bacterial, fungal, or parasitic, and could be bedbound for weeks. Various gastrointestinal maladies bedeviled her: reflux, malabsorption, pancreatitis.

Morgan Amanda was always underweight and pale, much more so as she grew older and her list of symptoms and accompanying medications grew longer. But she never stopped growing. At age twelve she shot up seven inches during a single school year, and was five foot nine at the end of seventh grade. By age fifteen she was just shy of six feet tall, and it became evident to her and her family that these varied symptoms were not separate issues, but probably part of a larger syndrome. The problem was that they didn't fit into any classic textbook illness.

Her parents took her on the first of several cross-country tours of specialists—from UCLA to Johns Hopkins—to figure out what was going on. Various diagnoses, surgeries, and treatment regimens came and went. Her list of pills lengthened. But her joints continued to ache and swell, and her energy level was nil.

Double vision, headaches, kidney infections, and bleeding ovarian cysts plagued her. Severe anaphylactic allergic reactions meant she had 911 on speed dial and epinephrine injections were stocked in her purse. Hand tremors and muscle weakness made gripping objects a challenge; four cell phones met their untimely deaths on the floor as a result.

By the time Morgan Amanda—now just over six feet tall and slender as a reed—arrived at Emory University, the working diagnosis was juvenile rheumatoid arthritis (RA). This inflammatory disease is famous for causing widespread and protean effects on the body, and could explain some of her strange conglomeration of symptoms. It wasn't a perfect diagnosis but it seemed to be the best answer that medical science could muster.

The simpler medications for RA weren't working and her doctors steadily ratcheted up the heft of her meds. Sometimes her symptoms were transiently alleviated, but always they returned. At the end of her sophomore year Morgan Amanda was receiving powerful immune modulators—intravenous gamma globulin and rituximab—that were infused like chemotherapy. She couldn't get them at her private rheumatologist's office because of her allergy to the latex gloves used there. The only place was at Emory, but because her rheumatologist was not part of the Emory system, he couldn't write the actual orders for the infusions. It fell to her primary-care doctor to write these orders.

Writing orders for chemotherapy-type infusions is not a mere technicality; it implies taking full clinical responsibility for big-gun treatment. Such treatments are generally the purview of specialists such as rheumatologists or oncologists, but Morgan Amanda's first primary-care doctor at Emory, who considered herself a bit of a cowboy, was willing to do it.

Happily, these treatments seemed to help. Morgan Amanda's symptoms were finally improving and her joint pains were calming. Less than a year into this treatment arrangement, though, her primary-care doctor moved to another state. Normally, when a doctor leaves, her patients are swiftly transferred to another doctor in the practice. But in this case no other internist at Emory was willing to assume Morgan Amanda's care. Her medical chart was intimidatingly dense. She had twenty-six diagnoses and was taking more than thirty medications. The list of meds to which she was allergic took up its own full page. She'd had seventeen major operations and had consulted with more specialists than anyone could count. On top of that there was the fraught issue of taking responsibility for the chemotherapy-type infusions.

Morgan Amanda was also strongly opinionated and ferociously well read on her conditions. She was majoring in health communication at Emory and was considering medical school, so handily mastered the clinical terminology and medical issues. She read medical journals avidly and researched her conditions thoroughly, and so came to the table with very definite opinions on the available treatments. Her sweet, friendly disposition and demure southern manners masked a steely resolve. She knowingly offered me the understatement that she's the type of patient who "arrives with baggage."

Depending on your vantage point, Morgan Amanda was either a "difficult patient" or an "empowered patient." Whichever the case, her medical condition was immensely complicated and would require an inordinate amount of work. No primary-care doctor wanted to take on this thankless task.

As one doctor after another declined her case, Morgan Amanda worried that she might be stranded without a primary-care doctor. Her mother in Chicago began calling the Emory Clinic administration, pressing the severity of the issue. The clinic director finally persuaded a doctor to take the case. Forty-eight hours later that doctor withdrew. The clinic director tried to persuade another doctor, who considered it, then turned it down because of the chemotherapy-type infusions.

The situation became so dire that the director himself had to temporarily assume medical care until a permanent doctor—one with enough experience and flexibility for this case—could be found. The desperate director finally turned to Juliet Mavromatis, a vivacious and energetic doctor with ten years of clinical experience, and begged her to take the case. Juliet was hesitant. Beyond the overwhelming clinical complexities of the case, the idea of taking responsibility for the infusions did not sit right with her. Not to mention that her practice was full and was officially "closed" to new patients. But she couldn't bear to see a patient abandoned. After some hesitation, she agreed to take this new patient into her practice.

I first encountered these two exceptionally smart and strong women when I was researching my previous book, *What Doctors Feel*. I'd been considering a chapter on friendship between doctors and patients, and so was trolling the Internet for relevant research or personal experiences. There wasn't much, but I did stumble across a blog that Juliet had written in which she touched upon the issue of "friending" patients on social media. I was on sabbatical in Israel that year working on the book, so I had several trans-Atlantic phone conversations with Juliet about the ethical and practical issues of friendships outside the clinical setting. In our conversations she mentioned one patient in particular—a patient with an extraordinarily complex medical history. She and the patient disagreed, often vehemently, about the treatment options, yet they also struck up something of a friendship. But Juliet was very careful not to reveal the patient's name or any particulars of the case.

Between phone calls I read more of Juliet's blog, and I noticed frequent comments posted by someone who was clearly a patient of Juliet's. The comments were cogent, thoughtful, and detailed. As I read through them I realized that this might very well be the patient Juliet had alluded to. From the nature and content of the comments, it was clear that this person certainly wasn't shy. She used her full name publicly and was openly sharing her own experiences. She offered advice and support to other patients but was also willing to reflect critically on herself.

I asked Juliet if she might convey a message to this person: that I was intrigued by the comments she'd posted and wondered if she might be interested in talking. Within days I received an enthusiastic letter from Morgan Amanda. She loved the idea of sharing her medical experiences, especially if there was something that might offer insights for others. Thus began a series of lengthy phone conversations, intricately scheduled to account for her college class schedule, her exams, and her numerous and far-flung medical appointments, as well as the time difference between Georgia and Israel. Some phone calls took place near midnight for me; others were early in the morning.

Coming from concrete Manhattan, I relished any opportunity to take in fresh air. The sun seemed to rise earlier in Israel, so for those early-morning calls, I'd drag a kitchen chair out into the yard and have our conversations while I sat under the *shesek* (loquat) tree, which was about as far as the phone reception would allow. And if I stretched my neck just so, I could catch a cerulean sliver of the Mediterranean Sea while we talked.

Morgan Amanda was an energetic and detailed storyteller. She remembered clearly how nervous she was at that first visit with Juliet on a humid Friday morning in early August. She was painfully aware that there were no other primary-care doctors willing to take her case. If she and this new doctor didn't connect—she couldn't even bear to contemplate what then. "I knew I was coming in with a reputation. I even dressed strategically to make a good impression," she recalled with a slight self-deprecating laugh. "But I felt stuck because I had no other options. I needed this to go well."

Morgan Amanda found the doctor to be nice, very professional, maybe somewhat shy. She gripped her copy of Virginia Woolf's *The Years* in her lap during the opening pleasantries, her long legs dangling nervously over the edge of the exam table.

Juliet recalled that first meeting going well. She found her new patient intelligent and pleasant. Juliet noticed the novel immediately, and Morgan Amanda mentioned that Virginia Woolf was her favorite author. When Juliet asked which of Woolf's books was her favorite, Morgan Amanda realized she'd stumbled upon a serious reader.

"*To the Lighthouse*," she replied, but added that *The Hours*—Michael Cunningham's homage to Woolf's *Mrs. Dalloway*—was also a favorite. Juliet had recently read *The Hours* in her book club. They quickly fell to discussing the intertwined narratives of Cunningham's novel, and how Woolf's characters transferred seamlessly to the present time.

Juliet liked Morgan Amanda's sharp wit and found that her pointed questions were stimulating rather than annoying. But they did have their disagreements. Juliet felt the combination of gamma globulin and rituximab infusions was overkill for her arthritis symptoms, which were under better control at the moment. More to the point, she wasn't convinced that RA was the diagnosis—or that RA was the *only* diagnosis.

Years before, one doctor had suggested offhandedly that Morgan Amanda might have a rare connective tissue disorder—either Ehlers-Danlos syndrome or Marfan syndrome. Morgan Amanda had even seen a geneticist by that time, but had been told that these illnesses were unlikely, and that in any case the available genetic tests weren't specific enough. Juliet seized on that, pointing out that a tall, lanky frame and history of eye problems were much more consistent with a connective tissue disorder than RA, and that she should consider pursuing genetic testing again.

Morgan Amanda found herself growing angry. It wasn't that she disagreed with the idea of genetic testing, but she felt she was being pushed to defend her illness to this new doctor. The fact that her symptoms were improved at this moment didn't mean she did not have RA. For a new doctor to make such a determination after just one examination seemed presumptuous. It was ignoring the complex clinical history in her chart. It was ignoring the fact that these "overkill therapies" might in fact be the very reasons her symptoms were currently in check. She sensed that Juliet was sizing her up as a difficult patient.

What makes a successful connection between doctor and patient when they first meet? Most patients seem to know it when they see it, even if they can't quite articulate the specifics. Before the visit is even over, most patients have a clear sense of whether this is a doctor they feel comfortable working with. But think about that for a moment. We would hardly buy a house or a car based on ten minutes of exploration. We wouldn't accept a job or make a financial investment with such scant information. Yet somehow we decide to invest our health in someone based on a single short encounter.

What is it that patients look for in doctors? When searching for a doctor, most patients still use word-of-mouth recommendations.[1] There is a plethora of doctor rating sites, as well as the many "quality measures" that are published online, but most people have trouble making sense of this jumble of information. This is partly because the data are disjointed. But mainly this is because most of us don't make decisions based on rational facts.

Decades of research by psychologists Daniel Kahneman and Amos Tversky has shown that humans do not act in the rational way that logic would suggest.[2] Patients may in fact research their prospective doctors' board certifications or mortality rates or blood-pressure control rates, but they don't necessarily use these numbers in choosing a doctor.[3] They tend to go with a doctor whom they feel they can trust.

In theory, this seems ridiculous—making a potentially life-and-death decision based on a gut feeling rather than facts. But when you examine it more carefully, there actually is a logic embedded in there. So much of the data—hard facts that they are—are free-floating and exist out of context. What does it mean that only 40 percent of Dr. X's patients with diabetes have their glucose under control? Well, it may mean that he does a terrible job with diabetes. Or it may mean that he has many elderly patients for whom "controlled" glucose might be harmful and so he appropriately allows their sugars to be higher.

Or it may be that he maintains a good relationship with those very difficult, complicated patients who can't or won't take their insulin. These are the kinds of patients who often bounce from one doctor to another. The fact that they stay with Dr. X suggests he's doing something salutary that maintains their trust. This keeps his patients engaged in the medical system but definitely makes his numbers look bad.

Perhaps Dr. Y, whose stats say that 80 percent of her patients with diabetes have their glucose controlled, is indeed a better doctor than Dr. X. Or maybe she is impatient with those who don't take their meds. The "difficult" patients find her off-putting and drift away, leaving her with patients who dutifully take their meds and furnish her with more-impressive numbers.

Does the surgeon with the lowest mortality rate achieve that sterling number because she's a technical genius or because she refuses to operate on patients with complex medical conditions? Is the doctor who is rated as "inefficient" a disorganized mess or does he spend extra time with each patient and so sees fewer patients per hour?

All of these "quality measures" simply measure what is easy to measure, and have only tangential connections to what is truly good medicine. So it may ultimately make sense that most patients do not make decisions about doctors based on these numbers. Most people want a doctor who is baseline competent, but most important, who will listen to them.[4]

The greatest fear of patients is that they won't be heard by their doctors and thus not get the medical care they need. From the get-go, it's not an even playing field and patients know that. They are aware that they are at a disadvantage when it comes to medical knowledge and experience. This is layered on top of the intrinsic power dynamics of a system that largely puts the doctor in control. Additionally, the whole interaction takes place on the doctor's home turf, not the patient's. The doctor gets the home-field advantage, at ease with the intricacies of the medical setting that, for most people, is only a few shades more alluring than an IRS audit. And of course it's the patient, not the doctor, who is doubled over in pain during the conversation, or who is nervously awaiting the CT scan report that will reveal whether the cancer has returned. All handicaps to the visiting team . . .

Then there is the time crunch, or should I say the time mismatch. The patient may have waited weeks or months for this appointment and so comes with a spreadsheet of accumulated concerns. He or she is desperate to pack every last issue into these precious few moments with the doctor. The doctor, on the other hand, is running late, is under pressure to be efficient, knows there is a pack of patients growing antsy in the waiting room, and has been given more work than can possibly get accomplished in the allotted time. Add to the mix a paper gown the heft of a Kleenex, plus the ambient temperature of Vladivostok in February, and you've got the perfect recipe for a potential disaster.

Patients sense that they have a singular and fleeting window to make their case—in terms of both actual minutes on the clock and legitimacy of illness. There is the need to convince an often-skeptical medical profession that they are really and truly ill, deserving of the doctor's time and of the medical profession's imprimatur of legitimacy. This is especially true of patients with vague complaints, especially if they appear outwardly healthy. Even Morgan Amanda, who had a five-pound chart documenting her ailments, found this a challenge because her symptoms didn't fit into any easy diagnostic category and because on the surface she looked relatively well.

Given the freighted nature of the initial doctor-patient meeting, the factors working against a smooth interaction, and all the competing tensions for both parties, it is almost astounding that this weighty encounter is mediated by the most rudimentary technology: a conversation. The physical exam and the subsequent tests do play a role, but the conversation between doctor and patient—the medical interview—is the single most important diagnostic tool in medicine. Not only is it the tool that yields the diagnosis, or at least focuses the path toward a diagnosis, but it is the tool that establishes the doctor-patient relationship, which is critical in the success of navigating medical care—something that Morgan Amanda and Juliet were quickly discovering.

So what happens when a doctor and patient talk? A typical interview, as it's referred to, begins with the doctor asking the patient the reason for the visit. This is the cue for the patient to begin his or her story.

I deliberately use the phrase "begin the story" because that is how most patients conceptualize their sense of becoming ill. Like any story, there is a beginning, middle, and end. There's a main character—the patient—and a definite plot (not to mention plenty of tension, conflict, and crises).

But this is not how it's traditionally viewed in medicine. The initial words of the patient are formally categorized as the "chief complaint." This chief complaint is the opener of the standard medical history and is meant to be a concise capture of the patient's main issue.

Already you can probably see the inevitable clash between doctor and patient. The patient has a story to tell and the doctor is scoping out a chief complaint. So it's not surprising that doctors typically interrupt patients within twelve seconds.[5] And it's not surprising that this is one of the biggest issues for patients. Being cut off is exceptionally frustrating because it makes clear that you aren't being listened to. It certainly isn't the most auspicious way to form a productive doctor-patient relationship and it's also a setup for medical error, but more on that later.

Morgan Amanda and Juliet navigated their new relationship, each eyeing the other somewhat warily. The patient wasn't sure if her new doctor was going to take seriously her illness and the importance of the gamma globulin and rituximab infusions. The doctor wasn't sure if the patient was going to be more work than she'd bargained for—someone who consumes vast resources of time and energy.

Morgan Amanda insisted she would be continuing the treatment recommended by the rheumatologist for her RA. She thought Juliet was being dismissive and somewhat paternalistic. But she kept the tenor of the conversation friendly and casual because she knew that she needed Juliet to write the treatment orders for the gamma globulin and rituximab infusions.

Juliet thought Morgan Amanda was being defensive and somewhat stubborn. But she kept the tenor of the conversation friendly and casual in turn because she knew that she needed to maintain a good working relationship with a patient who held strong—and controversial—ideas about her medical care.

After that first visit, Juliet reluctantly agreed to take on the role of prescribing the infusions. It did not sit well with her but it seemed that her patient had no other option.

Despite their disagreements over the infusion treatment, each found she rather liked the other as a person. They scheduled monthly visits because of the sheer enormity of the medical issues. At the beginning of each visit doctor and patient chatted easily, catching up on books they'd read, movie recommendations, schoolwork, Emory politics. It was only when they got to the infusions that they disagreed. There was tension between them as Juliet worried that this was a monumental medical mistake and Morgan Amanda worried that Juliet might back out at any moment.

Things went okay for the first few months. Then, during an infusion of gamma globulin in October, Morgan Amanda's body erupted in hives. Her eyelids, lips, and throat began to swell and very quickly it became difficult for her to breathe. As her blood pressure bottomed out, the staff quickly injected her with epinephrine and steroids, running large boluses of intravenous fluids into her IV. The episode of anaphylaxis slowly resolved, but now gamma globulin had to be added to her extensive list of life-threatening allergies.

In the months that followed, the swelling of Morgan Amanda's joints became more erratic and more severe. Her energy level plummeted, and there were days at a time when she was unable to get out of bed. Cooking, shopping, cleaning, and other household chores fell to the wayside. For someone who loved to read as much as Morgan Amanda did, the inability to read more than a page before her concentration flagged was spirit sapping. Despite her efforts, she could not keep up with her studies and finally withdrew from school for the semester.

That winter her mother moved from Chicago to Atlanta to help out. Her father commuted back and forth between the two cities. Though Morgan Amanda was immensely grateful for the assistance—she couldn't function without it—it was awful to be so physically dependent at age twenty-one and to know that she had uprooted her family. She nevertheless continued to insist on the rituximab infusions, about which Juliet continued to express reservations.

That April Morgan Amanda experienced another near-fatal anaphylactic reaction, this time to the rituximab. Another treatment had to be crossed off the list. Morgan Amanda was starting to feel desperate; would there be any medications left to help her? She had already plowed through every FDA-approved therapy on the market.

Morgan Amanda and her rheumatologist decided to notch up the treatment another level to cyclophosphamide—a chemotherapy agent used to treat lymphomas and serious autoimmune disorders. Juliet was vehemently opposed to this treatment. Cyclophosphamide is a ferociously potent drug—derived originally from the nitrogen mustard developed during World War I—and she worried that the toxicity would outweigh any benefit.

In general, Juliet didn't like being the "relayer" of another doctor's medical orders—there were too many confounding ethical, professional, and safety issues. But she had a personal aversion to this medication in particular. Many years before, when she was a resident, an attending had asked her to transcribe a set of medical orders for a patient with aplastic anemia. Among the complex cocktail of medications, there was one abbreviated "Cy." Juliet assumed it was cyclophosphamide, as this chemotherapy agent was used frequently on the oncology ward. In this case, however, Cy was meant to convey cyclosporine, a potent immune suppressant. Cyclosporine and cyclophosphamide are two of the heaviest sledgehammer medications in existence, and each one alone is approached warily by doctors. A medication error involving the two is about as nightmarish as it gets.

The patient received the wrong medication for several days before the error was noticed and rectified. Luckily, no significant harm had happened to the patient, but the potential for a devastating outcome was very real. The experience of being part of a medical error—the disclosure process, the reporting process, the self-examination, and the wrenching guilt—left a lasting impact on Juliet. Never again did she want to relay someone else's medical orders. Especially for cyclophosphamide!

But Morgan Amanda and her rheumatologist felt she needed more-powerful medications for her deteriorating condition, and cyclophosphamide was the only option. After much back and forth among all three parties, Juliet grudgingly agreed to write the orders and take on the responsibility for this treatment.

Predictably, the cyclophosphamide caused profound nausea and vomiting. After each monthly treatment, Morgan Amanda felt as though she'd been run over by a truck. It would take days until she could scrape herself out of bed. Her blood counts dropped and her hair fell out like any chemotherapy patient's. But after the second treatment her joint pain began to improve. Over the next few months the paralyzing morning stiffness began to recede and her energy slowly returned. Even Juliet had to agree—despite her reservations—that the treatment was having a salutary effect.

Morgan Amanda began to feel like herself again. She restarted her classes and was soon able to assume a full course load. Her twenty-second birthday came a few months into the treatment and she decided to celebrate. "I hadn't been sure I was even going to *make it* to twenty-two," she said, "and I wanted to thank everyone who helped me get there." She invited all the friends and family who had supported her, Emory professors and administrators she'd worked with, and also the medical staff, including Juliet. For Morgan Amanda, it was the chance to finally close the chapter on this awful year. The pages of the next chapter—crisp with expectation and promise—were waiting to be turned.

CHAPTER 3

It Takes Two

When I began writing this book I put out a call for stories about doctor-patient communication. Replies piled into my inbox but I quickly realized there was a fundamental problem. If the communication between doctor and patient had gone swimmingly, then there wasn't anything meaty to write about it. If the communication had gone poorly and there were issues that could be illuminating, usually one party was not interested in talking to me. Even in the research literature, many studies focused only on the patient's experience or, alternatively, on what the doctor had done.

Sonya Morgan, a researcher in New Zealand,[1] tried to square these two disparate viewpoints by videotaping a medical visit and then separately interviewing—and videotaping—the doctor and the patient immediately afterward. The most surprising result from a detailed review of all three videotapes was not so much that miscommunications occurred, but that both the doctor and patient were sometimes wholly unaware of the communication gaps.

In one case, a patient visited her general practitioner because of a mole. The doctor was concerned that it could be cancerous and referred the patient to a surgeon for prompt removal. When the video of the visit was reviewed, it was clear that the doctor had appropriately conveyed her concerns about the seriousness of the condition and the urgency of referral. It was also clear that the patient had understood this. A successful doctor-patient interaction.

When interviewed separately, both the doctor and the patient concluded that this had been a successful visit. The patient felt the doctor had listened to her concerns and responded appropriately. The patient also said she left the visit with a clear understanding of the doctor's recommendations. The doctor felt she'd done a good job both in terms of the medical issue and the communication with the patient.

But a week later the patient called the office to postpone her appointment with the surgeon. The doctor was surprised because she was sure the patient had understood the medical urgency of the situation. It also surprised the researcher who had independently observed that doctor and patient had communicated well.

How can such miscommunication, despite good communication, occur? Well, one thing to bear in mind is that each person in the conversation is knitted into his or her own backdrop of knowledge and experience, and all communication is filtered through that. The doctor, in this case, possesses an unambiguous understanding about the severity of skin cancer and the life-threatening reality should it turn out to be melanoma. These stark facts inform what she says to the patient and also inform her conclusion about how effective her words are.

The patient may have a very different understanding of the situation. Moles are common, everyone has them, they're part of everyday life. So although the doctor is saying how serious this mole could be and that removal is urgent, these words are filtered through—and possibly unconsciously diluted by—the patient's own experience and understanding. So although the patient understands and agrees with the doctor's recommendations, the ultimate meaning may settle in a different spot altogether.

How is meaning in communication created? It begins with the patient offering his or her primary reasons for a visit. However, these primary concerns or chief complaints are often quickly interrupted, as we noted earlier. Even if they are not directly interrupted in the true sense of that word, they are often "redirected" by the doctor within the first half minute of talking.[2] I know I'm just as guilty as the next doctor. The fear is that if I don't quickly hone in on the top priorities, the patient will ramble on ad infinitum and we'll never get through the visit. I don't think doctors are consciously trying to be rude, but time is always short and we need to get to all the important clinical issues (plus the many "quality measures" we are mandated to address). Ask any doctor and they'll tell you that in order to stay on time, you can't let the patient run on for too long. I knew one doctor who even ushered his patients straight onto the exam table upon entering the office so he could have the discussion part of the visit at the same time as the physical exam.

How long, I've wondered, would a patient actually talk if the doctor didn't say anything at all? I polled a few of my colleagues and they suspected two minutes for some, five to ten minutes for others, and a few said, "The entire visit!" One physician—a very empathetic and caring doctor—confided in me, "I know all the experts say you should let a patient talk uninterrupted at the beginning of the visit but it just doesn't work here. We'd be here till midnight!"

A group of Swiss researchers set out to find the answer to this question.[3] They examined the encounters of 335 patients at a university-based medical clinic in Basel. After the doctors asked their typical initial question (e.g., "What can I help you with today?") they were instructed not to say a single word until the patients completely stopped or specifically solicited the doctors to enter the conversation.

The average duration of the patients' monologues: ninety-two seconds. That was it—ninety-two seconds. Not exactly the deluge of historic proportions that most of us doctors fear. But, well, you know the Swiss—reserved, diplomatic, precise. Maybe Swiss patients lack the American gene for loquacious, self-referential gab. I decided to find out for myself.

The very next day after reading that study, I tried it out in my clinic. For every patient that day, I quietly clicked on a stopwatch right after I said, "How can I help you today?" The first patient took thirty-seven seconds, the second thirty-two. But these were basically healthy patients with only a few mild concerns. The third patient had more issues: unresolved back pain that was interfering with his job, plus glucose, cholesterol, and weight that were collectively creeping up to worrisome levels. He took a grand total of two minutes.

But then came the kicker, Josefina Garza. A lovely woman who used to be a teacher in her native Argentina, Ms. Garza was saddled with a vast array of disparate and insoluble pains, compounded by anxiety, depression, and irritable bowel syndrome, plus an elderly and demanding mother to take care of. Exactly the type of patient who can drown you with her list of complaints. Exactly the type of patient my colleague was referring to when she said that open-ended conversation "just doesn't work here." Ms. Garza is intelligent and personable; I love her droll observations about New York City's pretensions of culture, which of course can never measure up to the sophistication and elegance of Buenos Aires. But she was always in a lot of distress and our visits routinely ran overtime by orders of magnitude.

I could already feel the dread rising in me. If I let her talk uninterrupted, this visit would unfurl like a Borges labyrinth. I'd hear a dizzying list of symptoms from every organ system of her body, a rundown of her mother's medical ills, plus a stinging critique of the Metropolitan Opera's soulless production of *Turandot*. I wouldn't be able to provide any easy solutions for Ms. Garza's medical complaints and she would be frustrated with me and with her situation. I'd be forced into explaining the decisions of her mother's doctors as well as those of the artistic director at the Met who apparently routinely desiccates Puccini, not to mention the extortionate ticket prices that keep opera away from the masses, to whom it rightfully belongs, as it does in Argentina. Both of us would be in a sour mood by the end, and the whole thing would turn out to be a sprawling, onerous mess worthy of an atonal Schoenberg opera, which Ms. Garza, of course, would excoriate on philosophical grounds.

But I'd promised myself I'd let every single patient talk today without cutting anyone off. If I eliminated the "difficult" patients from my evaluation, then my data—however informal—would be flawed.

I heaved a sigh, girded myself for battle, and called Ms. Garza into the room. "How can I help you today?" I asked, and reluctantly clicked on the stopwatch

Her sigh was even heavier than mine. "Every single thing hurts," she said, "from my toes to my head." It was all I could do not to groan audibly, but I let her talk. I willed myself not to look at the stopwatch as she enumerated her concerns. Her left foot was aching. There were shooting pains in her gums. The tendinitis in her shoulders was acting up. Her scalp was painfully sensitive. Neck pain was radiating down her spine. Her mother had insomnia and was up at all hours of the night complaining.

Each time she paused, I asked gamely, "Anything else?" And there always was.

"I'm only forty-five," she said, knotting her fingers into her hair, "but I feel like I'm eighty-five. Every step hurts, and my head feels swollen to five times its size. It's like I'm walking through molasses."

I scribbled a few notes on paper as she talked but maintained eye contact with her the entire time, studiously avoiding looking at the computer screen—or the stopwatch. For good measure, I encouraged her to keep going. "Let's get everything out on the table," I said bracingly, "every last symptom and then we'll . . . then we'll, uh, we'll figure out where to go from there."

I let her keep talking, encouraging her to say more and more, until she had fully, truly, absolutely come to the end of all that she had to say. In the dip of silence that followed, I reached over to click off the stopwatch. I wanted to be discreet but my eyes couldn't resist slipping over to see what time it read. I had estimated that eight to ten minutes had transpired, but in fact it read four minutes and seven seconds. And the Met had come out unscathed. I suppressed the urge to say "Wow!"

Instead, I turned back to Ms. Garza and said, "Is this everything?" She nodded, and I showed her the list of all her concerns that I'd been jotting down. When viewed on the page it actually didn't seem so overwhelming. The list was long but it was finite. It seemed doable—to both of us.

Ms. Garza had already had a slew of MRIs and blood tests. She'd already been to a rheumatologist and a physiotherapist. We knew she didn't have lupus or rheumatoid arthritis or any electrolyte imbalance. We knew she didn't have anemia or hypothyroidism or B12 deficiency. I explained to her that she had *something* going on, some combination of a chronic pain syndrome and stress. "Medicine is very poor at explaining why and how these pain syndromes occur," I said, "but that doesn't mean we can't go ahead and start treating the symptoms."

We went down the list together, trying to identify which pains might be helped with ice packs, which might be helped with local heat and massage, which might best be treated with physical therapy, which might respond to pain medications. We talked about how antidepressants could be helpful and that seeing a therapist could decrease her stress. We discussed how she might get help in caring for her elderly mother. We discussed the critical role of exercise in treating chronic pain. And then we wrote up a plan.

At the end of the visit (which didn't run overtime by *too* much) she said something that I'd read about but had never heard a patient legitimately say: "Just talking about all this has actually made me feel better."

I wanted to jump up and sing an aria—which, luckily for all parties involved, I refrained from—but I was in the process of realizing something else. Just talking it all out had made *me* feel better. Like any doctor honest enough to admit it, I dread patients with chronic pain. Their medical visits are taxing and protracted. Usually the patient ends up dissatisfied and so does the doctor. This was the first time I'd ever had a visit with one such patient in which I'd felt *good* about it, like I was actually doing something to help, rather than just rearranging deck chairs. And I wasn't so worried now that another problem would spring out from left field and ambush me just as I was finishing the visit with Ms. Garza.

Of course, I can't attribute it all to the opening gambit of letting the patient speak uninterrupted, but I'm sure that it helped. I imagine that patients like Ms. Garza are accustomed to having walls erected in front of them. Their clinical issues can be so daunting that many doctors react—consciously or unconsciously—by attempting to turn off the spigot as expeditiously as possible. Perhaps the mere act of getting every last bit on the table made it seem less overwhelming and more manageable to Ms. Garza. It certainly felt that way to me.

Maybe it had to do with my being more receptive than I probably normally am. Maybe it was my tone being less pressured that lowered Ms. Garza's adrenaline level and relaxed the entire interaction. Maybe ignoring the computer and maintaining eye contact for the entire conversation changed what Ms. Garza was able to tell me. Maybe it was the sense of unlimited time that was the key element. Maybe it was simply admitting that passion and culture in New York could never hold a candle to Buenos Aires and leaving it at that.

We typically think of communication as the words exchanged when doctors and patients are seated across from one another at a desk during the "history" part of the visit. True, this is the bulk of communication and certainly the bulk of what communications researchers focus on, but over the years I've come to appreciate that a good deal of communication and connection arises during the physical exam. When I mention this observation, many people—both doctors and patients—are unconvinced. Who wants to chitchat after disrobing and having your body probed by a relative stranger in a room that feels like a meat locker? Who has time, anyway, for a real physical exam when there is so much to document in that electronic medical record and so little time?

So yes, there's less and less physical examination these days. Visits are shorter and competing issues wrench away precious minutes. The ease and temptation of CTs and MRIs, the constant fear of lawsuits, and—let's face it—the atrophy of our skills push doctors toward ordering more tests at the expense of a true physical exam. Often, the exam boils down to a halfhearted plop of the stethoscope on the fully clothed patient. I have been equally guilty of rushing through a pro forma physical exam when the pressure is on. And, in any case, the exam primarily serves as an adjunct to confirm or rule out a diagnosis that was ascertained in the history.

Doctors typically don't like to talk about their truncation of the physical because it stirs an awkward mix of guilt and longing within us. We recall wistfully our rounds as students, when our bow-tied and starched-coated attendings unhurriedly probed every fingernail, meticulously percussed the cardiac contours, palpated the epitroch-lear lymph nodes. We feel we are remiss with our current patients, that we are skimping on what has always been the sine qua non of the doctor-patient connection.

A decade ago people were predicting the permanent demise of the physical exam. Luckily there's been a resurgence of interest in the physical because it can obviate the need for many expensive tests.

In the past few years I've observed that the physical exam has taken on an important role again, though as a slightly different medical tool. Now that the computer is front and center in almost every doctor-patient encounter, doctors spend the bulk of the visit staring at a screen. Not only are our eyes yanked away from the patient, but our attention is fragmented by the disjointed and niggling nature of the typical computer interface. It's no wonder patients feel ignored by their doctors.

But then the doctor and patient move to the exam table and everything changes. This is often the first moment that we can talk directly, without the impediment of technology. We are physically closer to each other, actually touching. This is an intimacy, albeit of the nonromantic type, but an intimacy nonetheless. And all intimacies have the effect of changing the dynamics of an interaction. Obviously, there is a risk of changing it for the worse, but in my experience it is almost always a change for the better. Once a doctor and patient are at the exam table, touching, talking without the computer between them, conversation of a different sort is possible.

Countless times I have found that it is only during the physical exam that patients reveal what is truly on their mind. Whether it is the cough that they are reminded of now that I am listening to their lungs or the depression, eating disorder, or genital symptoms that they feel comfortable revealing once we are in a more intimate setting, there is something about touch that changes the dynamic.

So while the utility of the physical exam for diagnosing illness may not be quite as refined as it once was (though certainly still quite useful), it has become a tool of a different sort. These days, when I find that I'm at a communication impasse with my patient—we're disagreeing over something, or the patient just doesn't want to talk, or the computer is crashing, or the bedlam of my brain is threatening to erupt—I move instead to the physical exam. The messier the preceding crisis, the more time I take with the exam. The ritual and rhythm of the physical exam quell the din in my head and invariably I sense the patient relaxing as well. We pick up our conversation where we'd left off and now we are more focused, both on what we are saying and what we are hearing.

It is a refuge from the intrusion of technology, the intrusion of multitasking, the intrusion of assumptions and biases. It is a moment of *only* touching and talking. In the medical world—as in the world at large—there are precious few moments left of just touching and talking. As a diagnostic tool and as a therapeutic tool, this is irreplaceable. And we should not underestimate how much can be communicated in this moment.

———————

Medical training reinforces the idea that the more we doctors know, the better we can care for our patients. Residencies, fellowships, licensing exams, board recertification exams, continuing medical education courses, and medical journals all buttress the concept that sharpening our clinical knowledge is the key to excellent medical care. But there is a burgeoning field of research to suggest that this is necessary, but not at all sufficient. This is something that Marije Klein learned in the trenches.

Marije is a whirlwind of energy. Her effervescent laugh and engaging conversational style made her a popular TV journalist in the Netherlands, where she hosted a regional news show and covered health-care and human-interest stories. At thirty-eight, in the midst of her busy career and life with three young children, she was abruptly diagnosed with breast cancer.

Two brutal years ensued. First she had a radical mastectomy with reconstruction. The tumor was obdurate so radiation was required, plus a year of chemotherapy. Each of these then spawned their own complications: the radiation prolonged the healing of the mastectomy, and the chemotherapy required an indwelling catheter that triggered a life-threatening blood clot. The catheter had to be removed, making chemotherapy administration even more onerous. Implanting the prosthesis was yet another surgery. And of course there was the usual nausea, vomiting, dizziness, hair loss, poor appetite, lousy sleep, and generalized cruddy cancer feeling.

After the two-year ordeal things finally seemed to settle, and Marije felt she could breathe again. She had enough energy to help her daughter's class rehearse for the class musical, which would be performed on the night of her daughter's twelfth birthday. She and her husband began to plan a family trip to Croatia, their first vacation in years. First, though, Marije's brother and sister invited her to spend a long weekend at a friend's bed-and-breakfast in an Italian villa. It was the first time the three siblings had done a trip together, and there wasn't a place more conducive to post-illness recovery than Pietrasanta in Tuscany.

The villa was enchanting and the food delectable. On the first day of the trip, Marije's sister pointed out a stain on Marije's shirt. What might have been a spill of Chianti wine turned out to be serum seeping from Marije's surgical site. The chest wound had fissured open and rapidly became infected. Marije was rushed home and her doctor immediately hospitalized her. The prosthesis site was overwhelmed with infection and the prosthesis had to be removed.

With cancer's typical disregard for the human spirit, the surgery fell right on her daughter's birthday. Instead of attending the party and the class musical, Marije was flat on her back in an operating room as doctors dug out the prosthesis and the surrounding infected tissue. The planned family vacation to Croatia was flat on its back, too.

The surgery wasn't a panacea, though. After the operation, the wound refused to heal. Despite antibiotics and attentive nursing care, the wound wouldn't close, and thus began yet another unwelcome chapter in Marije's unwelcome cancer journey.

Open wounds are a challenge in any medical situation, but for someone who has had radiation that damages the surrounding tissue and chemotherapy that damages the immune system, healing can be arduous. Marije had to return, yet again, to the operating room to have the wound debrided and cleaned. Months of meticulous care followed—assiduous dressing changes, specialized bandages, topical antibiotics, biologic wound healers—but the wound remained stubbornly open.

After all the traditional approaches failed to heal her chest wound, Marije was referred for hyperbaric oxygen treatment, a procedure in which a patient breathes in 100 percent oxygen to maximally saturate the blood and tissues (ordinary air is 21 percent oxygen). Every day for nine weeks, Marije sat with nine other patients in a submarine-shaped tank that resembled a set from of a 1960s sci-fi movie. The sealed chamber was pressurized several times higher than normal air pressure, the equivalent of being about forty-five feet deep in the ocean. Patients strapped gangly oxygen masks to their faces. A few had to wear plastic globes over the head and neck, like cartoon space helmets. With the immense pressure bearing down all around them, they felt like they were deep-sea diving en masse.

Six weeks into the treatment, Marije had appointments with two of her doctors on the same day. One was the plastic surgeon and the other was Roel Straathof, the doctor supervising the hyperbaric treatment. The appointments were an hour apart, in offices lining the same hallway.

The surgeon examined the wound and saw that it was healing somewhat. But he shook his head regretfully: "This wound still needs surgery to close up properly."

Another operation? Marije was devastated. She'd already been through so many surgical ordeals by this point and was dreading another. "Is it really necessary?" she asked.

"Yes" he said definitively. "The surgery is necessary for the wound to close up properly."

Another operation! Marije spent the next hour digesting this crushing setback. Having already suffered complications from prior surgeries, she knew things could go wrong and that there was the very real possibility she'd end up worse than before—sicker, in more pain, even dead. She wasn't even forty years old and she felt like she'd already had a lifetime's worth of illness. But she'd known her surgeon for a long time and trusted his opinion. "I was so disappointed," she told me, "but I trusted this was for the best."

An hour later she dragged herself down the hall to her second appointment. Dr. Straathof had trained in general medicine and then went on to obtain a PhD in medical engineering. He enjoyed the application of the technical side of medicine to help patients who were often at the end of their rope. He recalls that Marije was a little hesitant about hyperbaric treatment at first, especially when she saw the bizarre-looking tank she would be inhabiting. But she was open-minded.

"I'd had a very long intake session with Marije when we first met," Roel recalled. "I was lucky that we'd had plenty of time to talk, so I knew about her goals as well as her fears, especially her fear of having another surgery. I knew which goals could be met by the hyperbaric treatment and which could not."

Roel took a look at her chest wound that day and smiled. "Well, that's coming along just fine," he said brightly. "Should be in good form by the end of the nine weeks."

Marije was stunned by his assessment. She told him that just one hour ago the surgeon had looked at the very same wound and said it wasn't healing properly, that she'd need another operation. Marije recalled that Roel nearly fell out of his chair with astonishment. "There's no need for further surgery," he said. "This will heal fine."

Marije remembered staggering home—confused, demoralized, and absolutely drained. How could this be? Here were two doctors whom she respected, whom she knew to be excellent. Yet they offered diametrically opposite assessments of her situation.

Roel had a slightly different recollection of the event. "In medical school we were taught that if you have to give a patient bad news, make sure you don't say anything else important afterward because the patient won't hear anything you say after the bad news. In this case, though, the reverse happened. I gave Marije the good news that she wanted to hear—that this wound will probably heal—but then she didn't hear anything I said afterward."

What Roel remembered telling her was that for the time being she didn't need surgery. But the wound could easily open up more, could get infected again, and if it had trouble healing again she would indeed require surgery. But he didn't think Marije heard any of that.

For Marije's part, she mulled over the contradictory assessment of her two doctors for several days and then made another appointment with the plastic surgeon. "Is it really necessary?" she pressed him. "Do I really need another operation?"

The surgeon didn't hesitate. "It's absolutely necessary," he said. "If you don't have another surgery it won't heal properly."

Marije rephrased her question. "What will happen if I *don't* have the surgery?"

The surgeon paused and considered. "Well, it will probably heal *eventually*, but there will be terrible scars on your chest."

At that moment, Marije understood. From the surgeon's perspective, if it healed with scars, it was not proper healing. He wanted her to have the best possible result, which in his eyes was a wound that healed with minimal scarring. But he hadn't really heard or understood what Marije wanted. After two years of treatments, complications, and infections, she just wanted to be done. She didn't care if there were scars crisscrossing her chest like the canals of Amsterdam. She just wanted the skin to close up so she could wear a prosthesis again. "I just wanted to walk around like a regular person and not look like a cancer patient," she told me. "I just wanted to be alive."

Roel had this assessment: "The surgeon and I ultimately told her the same thing, just in a different order. I told her that this wound will probably heal now but it could need surgery in the future. She just didn't hear the second part. The surgeon told her that the wound would need surgery, and then later—when pressed—told her that it would probably heal, though not in a pleasing way."

"During my career as a breast cancer patient," Marije later told me, "I've experienced some terrible listening: I have been called the wrong name. I have had doctors miss vital information I'm telling them. I've had nurses almost give me the wrong medication. But I've also learned that making assumptions is one of the worst things you can do as a doctor . . . and as a patient."

The surgeon had made an assumption about Marije, that she would prefer a less-disfiguring scar. It's certainly not an unreasonable assumption, but he didn't really hear Marije and understand her priorities. "What struck me most over my years of treatment," Marije said, "is how two people, a doctor and his or her patient, can sit in front of each other, talk to each other, but never get on the same level with each other."

After the back-to-back consultations Marije weighed the opinions of her two doctors, both of whom she held in high esteem. Ultimately she declined the surgery and opted to continue the hyperbaric oxygen treatment for a few more weeks. Slowly, slowly, the craggy edges of the wound began to knit themselves together.

"Both my doctors were right," she concluded. "It did heal *and* it healed with terrible scars." Marije, however, is okay with the scars. "It's very ugly," she said, with her trademark honesty, "but it's done. Now I can forget about the whole thing and just enjoy my three kids, my husband, my life." She also salvaged her ill-fated trip to Tuscany. Since her recovery she's organized annual writing retreats at the villa in Pietrasanta.

"With the gift of listening comes the gift of healing," wrote Catherine de Hueck Doherty. The Russian-born social worker, who became a leading voice in North American Catholicism, likely meant this in a spiritual sense. But as Marije Klein experienced, this is very much a concrete tenet of medicine.

CHAPTER 4

Now Hear This

Debra Roter, whom another researcher referred to as "the royalty" of researchers in communication, grew up in a working-class home in Flatbush, Brooklyn, in the 1960s. Her father was a butcher, and Yiddish was the lingua franca. Neither of her parents had graduated high school, though her mother later earned a GED. From these humble beginnings, Debra went on to create one of the definitive research tools for understanding how doctors and patients communicate.

Like most families of that era and locale, Debra's was mostly focused on the daily business of keeping family and livelihood going. Everyone was either an immigrant or the child of an immigrant, and noses were kept solidly to the grindstone. Debra recalled that when she first played Scrabble as an adult, she lost all the time because unlike her "American" counterparts, she'd had zero experience with board games in childhood.

But news and politics were a different story. Everyone took a visceral—and vocal—interest in the goings-on of the world. Political discussions and left-leaning newspapers competed with brisket, herring, and kugel for space at the dinner table. Debra's parents and three older brothers staked out opinions on everything; shyness in expressing such opinions was not a Roter trait.

One summer, after much begging and pleading, Debra and one of her brothers were sent to Camp Kinderland, the legendary summer retreat in the Berkshire Mountains founded by Yiddish labor activists in the early 1920s. Camp activities were saturated with social justice, progressive values, and lively horas. This being the 1960s, the counselors were usually busy coordinating protests at their colleges during the school semesters. Feminism was beginning to change the rules of the game.

Debra was steeped in these swirls of debate. Everybody, it seemed, was trying to say something. How it would all play out, nobody quite knew; but it was electrifying. In 1971, while Debra was attending college in California, the first edition of the feminist classic *Our Bodies, Ourselves* was published. This book had something to say that had not yet been heard before: women could be active participants in their medical care. This hardly seems like a radical statement today, but for all of the upheaval the 1960s brought to family, work, and society, the field of medicine was still firmly rooted in the hidebound 1950s.

The rigid medical hierarchy and the bedrock rules of doctor-patient interaction had hardly budged despite the foment in nearly every other aspect of society. The term "paternalism" wasn't even needed because the idea of the doctor telling the patient what to do wasn't seen as a problem. ("If our family doctor instructed my mother to crash my head through a plate-glass window," one of my colleagues recalled of that time, "she would simply have rolled up her sleeves and hoisted me through.") Telling the patient what to do was the very model of proper, effective, caring medicine. The idea that patients should speak up and assume an active role in their medical care, never mind try to be partners with their doctors in this care, was almost seditious. And, of course, nearly all the doctors were men. Even in 1970, fewer than 10 percent of doctors were women.[1] It wasn't until 1972, when the Title IX amendment to the Higher Education Act banned discrimination on the basis of gender, that women began entering medical school in significant numbers. (Currently, about one-third of doctors are women, though this percentage is destined to grow given that 47 percent of medical students are female.)[2]

Debra devoured *Our Bodies, Ourselves* and even today remains proud to have owned a 35-cent mimeographed copy of the original manuscript. The idea that language—how, when, and where we speak—could be a mechanism for women to assert power in a nearly all-male medical establishment was a heady thought. You didn't need money, position, or prestige to access some of that power; you just needed to understand how language and communication worked.

Debra's first job out of college was at the New York City Department of Health. Her task was to evaluate community health centers, to help define the needs of their patients. This involved talking with people in the community, understanding and prioritizing their concerns. One major issue was the low "show rate" to doctor appointments. At some inner-city clinics, fewer than half of appointments were kept. Debra thought perhaps that show rate could be improved if patients were more active in their care. Taking a page from *Our Bodies, Ourselves*, she encouraged patients to take a role in their care, even by doing something as elementary as planning a question to ask their doctor.

When Debra started her graduate studies in public health shortly thereafter, this idea became the central focus of her doctoral thesis. She hypothesized that if patients became more engaged in their medical care by asking questions, they would be more satisfied with the overall process and then keep their appointments more regularly.

So she set up a research project at an inner-city clinic in Baltimore near the Johns Hopkins campus, where she was working on her doctorate. The main thrust of the project was to have a health educator sit with patients for ten minutes before their appointments. The educator would ask about their medical conditions, which treatments they were getting, which medications they were on, and what they knew about side effects and prognoses. The educator would then encourage patients to come up with a few questions on these topics that they might ask their doctors. These questions were written down to be easier to remember during the visit. (For the control group, the educator simply reviewed the services that the clinic offered.)

Now, of course, Debra needed a way to figure out whether the patients actually asked the questions, so she audiotaped the medical visits. But then she was faced with transcribing three hundred audiotapes, word by word, onto paper in order to analyze what was being said during the visits. This was a laborious and daunting task. Plus, she was interested in more than just whether the patients asked questions. She was curious how doctors received the questions: With concern? Annoyance? Interest? Confusion? She realized she was interested not just in which words were being spoken, but rather in the whole gestalt of communication between the patient and doctor.

Debra wondered if there was a way to glean the crucial information from a conversation just by listening to the tape, rather than painstakingly transcribing every word that was spoken. There had to be a way to quantify what type of statement or question was being communicated and what sort of emotion was being expressed.

She realized she'd first have to figure out how to define a unit of speech. Would it be a word? A phrase? A sentence? Because she was interested in the meaning of what was being communicated, she decided the unit would be defined as a complete thought, whether that thought was a whole sentence, a small phrase, a single word, or even just an "mm-hmm" of agreement.

Then these units needed to be sorted out, or coded, into categories. First a unit would be coded as to who had spoken it, the doctor or the patient. Then it would be categorized by what purpose the speech was serving. For example, a good amount of speech in a doctor-patient visit is primarily about obtaining data, such as the doctor asking the patient about prior illnesses or the patient asking the doctor about lab test results. There's also "procedural" speech, directing a patient to, for example, sit on the table or take a deep breath. There is patient education and counseling, in which the doctor explains a test or how a medication works.

These categories were easy to identify because they are straightforward and don't vary much from visit to visit or person to person. Woven around these nuts and bolts of medicine, however, is an enormous amount of give-and-take that is less easy to define but is probably what patients are responding to when they say they have a fantastic doctor or a second-rate doctor. Or what doctors are talking about when they describe the most wonderful patient or the most difficult patient.

These elements of interpersonal connection can be hard to pinpoint and they can't be measured as easily as, say, whether doctors remember to introduce themselves at the start of visits (you'd be amazed at how many doctors forget to do this!). Various terms hint at this: bedside manner, compassion, enthusiasm, graciousness, warmth. A pure rationalist could say that they aren't really needed; if the patient is accurately diagnosed, treated, and cured, that's success. And from a statistical standpoint, that's true. A computer could surely accomplish any number of medical tasks, maybe even more accurately than a human.

But you can imagine—and maybe you have experienced—what medical visits *without* those components are like. Such visits leave much to be desired. When it comes to a medical visit that contains elements such as empathy, give-and-take, respect, and amiability—most of us know it when we see it, and surely know it when it's absent.

Debra was intrigued by these other elements in the doctor-patient interaction. She suspected these weren't just niceties that made the visit more pleasant but key elements in medical care. As a scientist, though, she needed a reliable way to measure these kinds of statements, something more than just "You know it when you see it."

So she created another category called "activation and partnership." These are statements from the doctor or patient that cue interest and connection, such as "Tell me more about that" or "So, what do you think?" or "Let me see if I've got this right. . . ." These types of statements clarify what's being said and, most important, let the speaker know that the listener is interested. As I would later learn from researcher Janet Bavelas, this is the doctor acting as a co-narrator with the patient, helping to draw out, enhance, and shape the patient's story. These statements ultimately end up doing double duty: establishing key facts for good medical care and also working to build a relationship between the two people speaking.

Then there are statements that signal emotional responsiveness. For instance, when the doctor acknowledges the pain of the patient's headache or the patient's frustration at having waited so long for an appointment. Or, conversely, the doctor might downplay the nausea or fatigue caused by a medication. These are statements that indicate how the person is responding to the other person's concerns and serve to legitimize—or minimize—what the other person is saying.

Within these broad categories, the units of speech had to be subcategorized as to whether they were questions, statements of opinion, statements of approval, or requests for clarification. There were also categories for statements of agreement, personal comments, and requests for questions. Questions could be open-ended or closed-ended. In the end there were several dozen distinct types of speech that took place in the conversation of a typical medical visit. Debra now had a detailed system for categorizing the myriad elements of doctor-patient communication.

On top of all these detailed categories of speech, Debra added one more thing to be recorded: the emotion being expressed. It was critical to know whether a statement was spoken matter-of-factly, irritably, sympathetically, angrily, or anxiously. The measurement of emotion was a crucial addition to the system. In the old-fashioned transcribing system, there would be no way to distinguish one doctor's warm, friendly "How are you?" from another's curt and perfunctory "How are you?"—even though these obviously set the stage for radically different communication. This additional category rated the emotional temperature of what was being said.

Collaborating with Judy Hall, a faculty member from her dissertation committee, Debra had now created a scientific way of measuring both the factual content and emotional components of conversations between doctors and patients.[3] Rather than having to transcribe on paper every word that was spoken, Debra could listen to the tape and simply check off the appropriate categories for each unit of speech that occurred. In the end she would have a detailed analysis of each conversation. She could know, for example, how many empathetic statements a doctor made, or what percentage of the visit was spent gathering data, or how many questions a patient asked, and then cor-relate these numbers with medical outcomes such as blood pressure control or medication adherence. Because these were hard numbers and not simply impressions of what had occurred, statistics could be applied to rigorously evaluate the outcomes.

For Debra's original study about patients asking questions of their doctors, this coding system enabled her to document that the ten-minute session encouraging questions actually worked. It turned out that these patients asked twice as many direct questions as patients in the control group.[4] On average, the patients asked two questions per visit, as opposed to one question for the patients in the control group. Doesn't sound like much of a difference, but the patients who asked the extra question were 17 percent more likely to keep their follow-up appointments. That's an effect that's noticeable and meaningful.

Unexpectedly, however, the patients who asked more questions left the medical visit with more anxiety and anger. Overall, they were *less* satisfied with their experience. This ran counter to Debra's hy-pothesis, that once patients were more active in their health care they would be more satisfied.

This outcome was puzzling but it did have a paradigm in the po-litical upheavals of the day. When historically passive segments of society—women, African Americans, immigrants—began speaking up, the traditional order of things was challenged. The establishment wasn't necessarily pleased to have the comfortable working order destabilized. Reactions and backlashes made things worse, and it often took years or even decades before society settled around new norms—if it ever did. Patients in the 1970s—especially patients from lower socioeconomic strata—were generally a docile group. Doctors told patients what to do and that was that. One can imagine that having patients question this would be a surprise to doctors at the very least, or perhaps an affront or even an insult. It could change the tenor of the interaction and leave both parties feeling uncomfortable.

Or it could simply be that doing anything different than usual inherently feels uncomfortable. The patients had been asked about their satisfaction directly after the visit, and may have felt out of sorts from the experience of stepping out of their comfort zone moments earlier. But the fact that their show rates six months later were higher suggests that they may have grown more comfortable with this type of interaction. Although the patients weren't specifically polled again after six months, they may have indicated their increased satisfaction by voting with their feet and returning for the next appointment.

The bigger question for Debra Roter was how all of this affected medical care. Now that she had a tool to rapidly and reliably measure how doctors and patients communicated with one another, her career was ready to unfold. The tool became known as the Roter Interaction Analysis System (RIAS), and it has become the standard yardstick in communication studies.[5] It's been used in every aspect of medicine. Debra herself has published more than two hundred papers using the system to study communication in the fields of oncology, podiatry, pediatrics, obstetrics, psychiatry, and geriatrics. She has used the RIAS system to research medication adherence, sexually transmitted diseases, diabetes, domestic violence, genetic testing, HIV, hypertension, Alzheimer's disease, asthma, malpractice, the prescribing of psychiatric medications, the teaching of communication to medical students, the use of humor, the effects of patient race and ethnicity, and the role of doctor gender. It's been used in Japan, Israel, England, and China.

The term "medical visit" is often used in a way that suggests it is a very standard thing, that doctor-patient encounters are generally homogeneous. Debra and her colleagues suspected that there was more variety, and that the different types of encounters presaged different outcomes. They analyzed more than five hundred medical visits in ordinary clinics and private practices.[6] These were ongoing-care visits (that is, not new visits) between 127 doctors and 537 patients. These visits are the bread and butter of general medical practices. Most patients in these visits have a couple of chronic conditions to check in on and an occasional new issue to discuss. Then there are clusters at either end of the severity spectrum—some patients with multiple, serious conditions, and some who are generally healthy, just coming for an annual checkup.

By examining the communication between patients and doctors, the researchers were able to divide these encounters into several types of visits. The first was the traditional medical visit, which they termed "narrowly biomedical." As the name suggests, nearly everything in this type of visit was about medical issues. Neither the doctor nor the patient delved into psychological or social issues. Much of the doctor's talk involved asking questions of the patient, usually of the closed-ended variety. (Have you ever had chest pain? Do your legs swell? Do you get dizzy?) About one-third of doctor-patient visits were of this "just-the-facts-ma'am" type.

Another one-third fell into the category of "expanded biomedical" visit. This visit was still predominantly medical in nature, with the doctor asking the lion's share of questions, but the doctor and patient did venture into some of the psychological and social wellbeing of the patient.

The elements were far more balanced in what was called the "bio-psycho-social" category. Patient talk was equally divided between the medical and the psychosocial. Physician talk was still weighted toward the medical but much less so than in the other categories. One-fifth of visits fell into this category. (In a sprinkling of visits, the patient talk was nearly all psychosocial.)

Far fewer visits fell into what the researchers termed the "consumerist" category. Here the patient was more like a customer utilizing a service, in this case the doctor's medical knowledge. The patient asked most of the questions and the doctor spent the visit dispensing information. Little of the psychosocial realm came up. These were about one-tenth of visits.

When asked their opinion about the visits they'd experienced, patients were distinctly unenamored of the narrowly biomedical visits. These had the lowest satisfaction ratings. Patients preferred the more balanced experience of the bio-psycho-social visit. These visits were more evenly balanced not just by topic but also by who did the speaking. Interestingly, doctors were not especially fans of the narrowly biomedical visits, either. They ultimately saw these visits as inefficient, making poor use of their time and yielding low-quality data.

One analysis in the study that intrigued me was of communication control, that is, who feels in control of the conversation. Not surprisingly, patients felt they had the least control of the conversation in the narrowly biomedical visits and had the most in the consumerist visit, where they asked the questions and the doctor served mainly as the consultant.

The term "consumerist" has always rubbed me the wrong way— the whiff of shopping-mall abyss is enough to make me cringe—but I know exactly what kind of visit this is. The patient arrives armed with questions and I am already on the defensive even before the patient has opened his mouth. When the patient unfolds the shopping list of questions with that crisp, disheartening snap, immediate pangs of dread besiege me.

When I've thought about why my hackles get automatically raised, I've usually chalked it up to the volume of requests that typically follow and the impossibility of addressing everything in a short visit. But Debra's study made me wonder if I'm perhaps reacting unconsciously to the ceding of control. In more-typical visits, the patient brings up a few things and then—if I look honestly at myself—I take over the conversation. I rapidly prioritize the issues and then start asking the questions that eventually dictate our course of action. Of course I am engaging the patient in all of this conversation, but the truth is that I'm usually steering the course. When the patient begins by positioning herself as the asker of questions, as in the consumerist type of visit, the dynamic changes. Maybe that's why I feel uncomfortable.

When I look back at what I just wrote, I notice that I said the patient comes "armed" with questions. Indeed, I sometimes feel like I'm under attack when the barrage of questions comes forth, along with the expectation that there will be ready answers for every one. Part of my defensiveness is surely that I know that I will disappoint for a good percentage of these questions. Medicine is much less precise than we'd like to think, and so when that sheet of questions unfolds, I know I'll be equivocating—and disappointing—quite a bit. My patients will be annoyed, as will I.

Reexamining my reactions through the prism of this research is helpful. No one relishes losing control and we all respond to this—usually unconsciously and often negatively. Next time I notice a reflexive spine-stiffening when a patient unfolds a list of questions, I'll try to remind myself that the center of control is going to shift a bit. If I can readjust myself in advance, maybe I won't lose my balance so easily.

One of the (many) things Debra Roter is using her RIAS system for is to help train doctors to use communication more effectively. A standard method many medical schools use is the videotape review. Medical students or residents are videotaped interviewing patients and later review the tapes with a faculty member. At our medical school I participated in this for years, but I have to admit that I found it painfully laborious. I would sit with four students and we'd watch a few minutes of one tape, then discuss it. Then we'd watch a bit more and offer a few comments. But we could never watch the full visit because it would take too long, plus so much time was wasted rewinding and fast-forwarding. In the end, we'd glean only a little from the experience. The juice never felt worth the squeeze.

"With RIAS," Debra explained, "you can look at the entire visit at once." An intern could see that she had offered reassurance to the patient seventeen times but never once made a statement that offered empathy, even though the patient had raised ten issues of concern during the conversation. Furthermore, the intern could click on those seventeen "reassurance statements" and listen to what she'd actually said. She might find that she used the same phrase—"There's nothing to worry about"—over and over, which probably began to sound like a platitude to the patient. She could click on the nine "patient concerns" and realize that the patient had only two real concerns but kept repeating them because the intern kept saying, "There's nothing to worry about."

A medical student could see, for example, that he was speaking for 80 percent of the time while the patient spoke only 20 percent of the time. He could be gently reminded to cede the floor more frequently.

Most doctors have never had their conversations with patients analyzed, and I bet many of us would be surprised to learn what we look like and sound like. The first time I saw myself on videotape I was shocked to see how much I talk with my hands. I was a veritable tarmac flag-waver. It's a wonder I didn't accidentally knock any patients off the exam table.

I also noticed that whenever I was asked a question for which I had to stop and think, my eyes would flit up toward the ceiling and hover there while I cogitated. This, I know, is common behavior, but it still annoyed me to see my gaze wander off. However, when I was really stumped, I would actually close my eyes completely. Seeing that on tape horrified me. Did my patients think I was zoning out completely? Did they think I was running low on caffeine or maybe debating what to make for dinner that evening? Either way, seeing these tapes made me more conscious of how I was responding to my patients.

Simply having this enhanced consciousness may be sufficient to increase the effectiveness of communication. If patients recognize, for example, that they aren't asking their doctors enough questions, they may be able to focus the conversation to ensure that their most important concern is addressed. If doctors notice they're dominating the conversation or ignoring issues beyond the strictly medical, they may find that a few small adjustments will increase their effectiveness, as well as the satisfaction all around. David Baron and Tracey Pratt are one such doctor-patient pair who made the effort to be more conscious of their interaction, and it propelled them onto an unexpected path.

CHAPTER 5

With All Good Intentions

When Tracey Pratt gets an idea in her head, she goes for it. So when she decided, after five years as a schoolteacher in Washington, DC, to head north for graduate education at the age of thirty-eight, she simply packed up and moved to Cambridge, Massachusetts. Everyone knows that's where the good universities are, and she'd iron out the details later. She figured, "I can teach anywhere, so let me get a job in Cambridge and then start applying to programs."

Tracey has that combination of no-nonsense directness and easygoing warmth you might expect of someone who teaches middle school and lives to tell the tale. Her demeanor is both crisp and engaging, but there is also a good dose of self-deprecating humor that hints at why she is so successful with the preteen set. She is also very confident. Indeed, after her very first (and only) job interview, she found what seemed like a perfect match—as a sixth-grade special education teacher in a school that embodied her educational philosophy. The job offer came through before she'd even made it back to her hotel room, and she was thrilled.

That first year was challenging—fun and exciting—but also stressful. Adjusting to a new classroom and a new school system, even a good one, is never easy. She didn't know anyone in town and her family was far away. Her stepfather in Florida passed away that first Thanksgiving and it was hard being so far from home. Cambridge was a lovely town—but, oh, those winters. The worst part, besides trudging to the bus stop through mounds of snow and slush, was that the sun disappeared by 4 p.m. The whole winter seemed submerged in darkness.

By the end of that first school year, Tracey was exhausted. Juggling a classroom of sixth graders is never for the faint of heart and this year was no exception. Even though she loved her work, navigating a new city, a new job, and a new life had taken its toll. To top it off, a powerful heat wave had settled over the Boston area that June—the kind that makes you pine wistfully for the three-foot snowdrifts of January. The last few weeks of June dragged on and her goal became just to finish out the school year. Like every other inhabitant of Cambridge that June, Tracey was permanently hot, tired, cranky, and thirsty. Pepsi was her drink of choice, and she consumed it constantly to stay cool. Unfortunately, this also caused her to run to the bathroom all the time, which made her even crankier.

One Saturday toward the end of the month the heat had become more than she could take. No matter what she did she was hot and draggy. Finally, she gave up trying to grade assignments and picked her way through the sticky afternoon to go to the movies at Boston Common. Anything to cool off. The air-conditioning was on full blast and her extra-large Pepsi was a veritable arctic ice floe, yet she left the theater feeling hotter and thirstier, if that was even possible. The next day she was too tired even to go to church, which had always been an ironclad part of her life.

When Tracey spoke to her mother that night and described how she was feeling, her mother replied matter-of-factly, "Sounds like you have diabetes. Go see a doctor."

"I do not have diabetes," Tracey snapped. "No one in our family has diabetes. I just need this school year to end and this heat wave to finish already!"

Monday morning was like moving through hot tar. It took Tracey forever to get ready for work. It was all she could do to put one foot in front of the other as she walked from the bus to school in the thick heat. Even letting her arms swing alongside her during the walk seemed arduous. "I realized then," she said, "that I really needed to see a doctor."

She called the doctor's office and described her symptoms to Marva, the nurse. The first thing Marva asked was, "Do you have diabetes?"

"No, I do not have diabetes!" Tracey shot back. It was like a conspiracy, it seemed, for everyone to assume she had diabetes. Tracey arrived at the clinic as soon as the school day ended. Marva immediately pricked her finger to check her blood sugar. The glucometer wasn't able to register a reading. "Maybe it's a misread," Marva said. "Let's try again."

They did a finger-stick a second time but the glucometer still wouldn't register a reading. "Maybe this machine isn't working right," Marva said. She left the office and returned with a second glucometer. Again, a reading wouldn't register. "Let's check your urine instead," Marva finally said.

That was probably the one task that didn't require effort for the exhausted Tracey, as the Pepsi-urine pipeline was operating in full waterfall mode. Minutes after Marva took the urine sample she returned to say, "You definitely have diabetes. The glucose is so high that we can't even get a reading! That's why the glucometer couldn't give us a number. It's so high that we might even need to hospitalize you right now."

Tracey's first reaction was a panicked Oh-my-God-what-am-I-going-to-do? "I felt like I was in an immediate crisis," she recalls, "and I guess I was." A tube of blood was quickly drawn for *stat* labs in order to figure out whether hospital admission would be necessary. Tracey sat in the waiting room while the blood test was being run, wrestling with this new concept of having diabetes. Was she now going to be someone who was sick? Who was disabled? Would she be forever defined as a diabetic? At least the waiting room was air-conditioned, even if the "stat" blood test took two interminable hours.

"I began to cry while I was sitting in the waiting room," Tracey remembered. "I felt helpless." She called her mother and told her the news. Her mother reassured her that everything would be fine but began wondering aloud if she had been remiss in Tracey's medical care in childhood. She recalled several times that Tracey had felt faint as a teenager and wondered if she'd somehow missed something.

As Tracey wrestled with these thoughts and emotions, an older man in a wheelchair rolled by. Her teaching-mode pragmatism switched abruptly into gear. Diabetes wasn't a disability, for goodness' sake. It wasn't incapacitating. She had kids in her class who managed their own diabetes. If sixth graders could do it, she could surely do it. She would just do what she needed to do and then get on with her life. She decided then that diabetes would neither run her life nor ruin her life.

She had to hang tight onto that sentiment, though, because the first words out of Marva's mouth when she returned were "You better call your mother and thank her. Had you waited another day, you would have come here by ambulance!" She gave Tracey a shot of insulin to rapidly lower her blood sugar, and so began a new chapter of Tracey Pratt's life.

"She was likeable right off the bat." That's how Dr. David Baron described Tracey. David is an internist in his midfifties with a low-key style and contemplative nature. Despite having spent the past twenty-five years in and around Boston, his voice retains the studied inflection and pacing of his rural Ohio childhood. He was first exposed to the possibilities that medicine offered when, at age twenty, he volunteered for a summer in the Dominican Republic. He and his team tramped along the steep banks of the Ozama River, vaccination tools in tow. People there lived in shacks made of plywood, tin, and palm fronds. There were no streets, no addresses, no medical records of any kind. Community members simply lined up when the medical volunteers arrived, and the team went down the line, vaccinating everyone in one fell swoop.

David recalls being awed by the potential impact that medicine could have. In one morning, an entire neighborhood could be vaccinated against diseases that were otherwise fatal. After college he joined the Peace Corps and returned to the Dominican Republic to continue working with this community. One day, he was returning home to the small village where he was living when he heard a cry for help. A man was having a seizure in the middle of the road. Everyone turned to David with expectation—he was the American, after all, the person with a college education. They assumed he would "do something." But of course he didn't have any real medical training— he was just a skinny white kid from a small town in the Midwest. David watched, helpless, guilty, as the man's seizure ran its course. The man's body eventually quieted and he was okay, but David felt chastened by his lack of skills and inability to do anything practical. Medical school offered the promise of that practicality, and David jumped eagerly in that direction.

After completing his medical training, David found a job in Cambridge. He was attracted to the Cambridge Health Alliance because of its commitment to community medicine, to the everyday working folks of Cambridge, to underserved populations often lost in the shuffle, all while maintaining the rigorous academic standards of a Harvard-affiliated teaching institution.

"It's hard to get to know a patient fully in a fifteen-minute visit," David said, "but when I first met Tracey I thought, 'This will be easy; she's a teacher! I love teachers. Surely she'll strive to be the best student.'"

For Tracey, the Cambridge Health Alliance was a matter of convenience. She chose it when she arrived in the city because it was right in her neighborhood and it didn't matter to her whether it was a clinic or a private office. Her life was busy and she was completely healthy so she didn't have any need to be choosy when selecting a place or doctor for her health care. In fact, the reason she picked out Dr. Baron from the list of doctors was because his name was the easiest to pronounce. Before the diabetes diagnosis, Tracey and David had met maybe once, for some minor ailment that neither even remembers. But now, with the diagnosis of a serious lifelong illness, they were abruptly joined together as though they were in a three-legged race. There hadn't been time for advance planning or forethought, and now they had a marathon to run together.

David remembers that at first Tracey seemed a bit shy, with a hard-to-crack exterior. He sensed she was feeling him out. Could she trust this doctor? Would he really understand her? He was well aware that the stakes were high. The potential downsides to diabetes are well known and grim: heart attacks, kidney failure, dialysis, amputations, blindness. Diabetes is rarely a "gratifying" illness for doctors *or* patients. There are no easy or dramatic treatments, no equivalents of antibiotics routing out pneumonia, or a heart transplant granting a new lease on life. There is only the endless slog of giving up foods you always loved, of doctors haranguing about losing weight, of never-ending blood tests, of side-effects-laden medications that are only modestly effective, of expensive supplies that are rarely covered by insurance.

The disease being so common, David had enormous experience treating patients with diabetes and knew the gamut of outcomes. There are always a few patients who—whether because of genetics or grit or a more malleable variant of the disease—are easily able to corral their diabetes under control. These patients seem to be able to turn their lives on a dime, effortlessly shedding a lifetime of starchy diets and sedentary behavior. They seem to thrive on quinoa and kale, never pining for the white rice and doughnuts of their youth. They somehow manage to find an hour a day to spend on the treadmill, losing thirty pounds without much struggle. No matter what their doctors do or don't do, these patients thrive.

On the other end of the spectrum there are some patients simply unable to face the reality of diabetes. These patients ignore their disease and their medical care until they end up in the emergency room requiring dialysis or foot amputation or bypass surgery. No matter what their doctors do or don't do, these patients end in a blaze of irreversible medical complications.

But the vast majority of patients exist in the middle ground, trying their level best to deal with a frustrating illness and a society of supersized sodas that seems determined to thwart their efforts. David knew that of all the tools in the medical armamentarium, a strong and trusting doctor-patient relationship was one of the most powerful. Some argue that it is *the* most powerful. Certainly for a long-term illness with frequent setbacks and ongoing frustrations, a solid connection is critical.

David recognized that the connection he and Tracey would ultimately forge could have major medical consequences—positive and negative—not to mention determine whether their visits together would be pleasant, awkward, fractious, or vexing. A thoughtful person by nature, David turned this over in his mind for some time, contemplating how best to cultivate a working relationship with Tracey.

For Tracey, the first few weeks after the diagnosis were rough. She had been hoping that her new metformin pills would make her feel "normal" again, but instead they just gave her diarrhea. It took months for her body to adjust, but eventually it did. After opening up her garbage pail and tossing in all of her pasta, white bread, and sugar on that first day, Tracey made an effort to improve her diet. But it was hard. Really hard. Preparing healthier meals took more time and more planning. Vegetables were always going bad in the fridge and had to be thrown out. The Pepsi had to go. Salads were okay, but only okay; they weren't especially beckoning or satisfying, and she had to make a conscious effort to eat them. Tracey forced herself to start eating breakfast in the morning, something that wasn't a natural for her body. Intellectually, she knew it was the healthy thing to do but that didn't make it any more palatable. Plain oatmeal with dried cranberries was about the only thing she could stomach in those early hours.

The hardest time of the year was the carbo-clysmic gauntlet that stretched from Thanksgiving to New Year's. You couldn't squeak two feet down the linoleum school corridors without running into a plate of doughnuts or a bag of chocolate-covered pretzels or a vat of caramel corn the size of an oil drum that someone had lugged in from a big-box store in the suburbs. Leftover pumpkin pies and apple pies showed up in the teachers' lounge. There were bowls of chocolate Kisses in the principal's office and candy canes taped to any surface that wasn't plastered with tinsel or book reports. Extra cupcakes from class parties piled up on the counters of the main office. Grateful parents brought in pastries. Students gave teachers chocolates from Taza or L. A. Burdick in Harvard Square. Colleagues baked homemade Christmas cookies to share with their coworkers.

On top of that sugar haze baseline were the holiday parties that started at Halloween and ran more or less continuously until mid-January. It was as though American society had conspired—under the auspices of peace on Earth and goodwill toward men—to doggedly challenge the nutritional resolve of every diabetic from Cambridge to Bethlehem itself.

Diabetes turned out to be like an annoying houseguest who never left. It was everywhere—in the food you bought, in the meals you prepared, in the monthly trips to the pharmacy, in the prices of meds that weren't fully covered by insurance, in the temptations that beckoned on a daily basis, in the inner debate that played out for every morsel of food you consumed, in the idea that maybe you weren't as healthy as you thought you'd been, in the idea that evolution had designed your metabolism to cling onto every last fat cell and carb just in case an ice age was hovering around the next corner to devastate the planet's food supply.

What Tracey hated the most, though, was pricking her finger to check her blood sugar. It was awkward, it was painful, it took up precious time and mental energy in an already busy day. But the worst part was that it could show you—in stark digital numbers—how awful you were doing, despite all the hard work and medications.

In the three years that followed, Tracey's life became even busier. In addition to teaching she became very involved in her new church. She was a staple at the many church events but found her calling in liturgical dance. This was a way to interpret God's word via dance, using gospel music and biblical text, and she turned out to be a natural. Tuesday nights were packed with dance sessions and Bible study, which she volunteered to teach. Even though it was on a school night, she was willing to stay up late for these activities. She spent hours during the week preparing for each Bible study class, which she found endlessly fascinating and enjoyable. "In fact," she confided to me, "I daresay that I enjoyed planning for and teaching Bible study more than I enjoyed planning for and teaching math." Ever the diplomatic teacher, she summed it up this way: "For me God comes first. But math is a close second!"

The civic life of Cambridge came in as a close third. Tracey plunged into local politics, organizing meetings, strategizing for local campaigns, and canvassing for signatures to get candidates on the ballot. As a volunteer for the Democratic City Committee, she was the interface between the Democratic Party and the community. Her hard work drew praise and she was selected to attend state conventions and be part of larger civic committees.

Tracey tried to keep a realistic view on the diabetes. A wonderful nutritionist offered the perspective that there wasn't really a "diabetic diet" that she needed to follow—just a balanced diet of healthy foods with everything in moderation. And she also managed to avoid the trap of obsessing about weight.

"Weight for me was never much of an issue," she told me, "but Dr. Baron would definitely comment if I gained a few pounds, letting me know that I would have many more difficulties if I gained weight." Ironically, she got the opposite reaction from her church friends: "People in the African American community would say that they didn't understand why I had diabetes because I was too 'skinny' to have diabetes. In their experience, most people who develop diabetes in adulthood were much more noticeably overweight."

Exercising wasn't as much of an obstacle for Tracey as it is for some people. She loved the liturgical dance she was learning and often found herself practicing the moves in her kitchen, which was the biggest room in her tiny, basement Cambridge apartment. She'd run track in high school and college so didn't mind going to the gym, but finding the time to do so was a Sisyphean task. She was so busy that there wasn't enough physical space on her calendar to squeeze in all of her commitments. There was hardly time for proper grocery shopping or preparing healthy lunches in advance. She was juggling so many things that it was hard to remember to get her medications refilled before they ran out. Getting to the doctor during regular business hours was nearly impossible.

"It was pretty easy to cancel a doctor's appointment if it conflicted with something else on my schedule," Tracey said. And there was always something else on Tracey Pratt's schedule. She took her medications—most of the time—and checked her blood sugar some of the time. But things were always getting in the way. There were papers to correct and parents to call. There were meetings for school, and for her church group, and for the Democratic City Committee. There was Bible study preparation and dance class. There were events to plan, events to attend. And there were always her students—lovable, stimulating, but with endless needs. As her doctor, David worried. Tracey's blood sugar level—though lower than it had been initially—remained persistently elevated, and this put her at increased risk for all of the dreaded complications of diabetes.

"She'd accept some of my recommendations," David recalled, "but ignore others." More than many doctors, David was the type who invested his soul in his medical practice. He so much wanted Tracey to succeed. Unlike many of his other patients, Tracey was educated and had a full-time professional job; she was responsible and organized. David knew she understood his medical recommendations—so why did she ignore so many? Did he need to try harder and schedule more frequent visits? Or maybe he needed to pull back and give her more space. Success seemed to be within their grasp, yet it kept eluding them. It was heartbreaking.

Tracey had a slightly different take on things. "We weren't seeing eye to eye," she told me. "No matter what medical issue I went to him for, the conversation *always* went back to diabetes and me not taking care of myself. I mean, I could go there for a pulled muscle in my back or a mammogram question, and it was all about my blood sugar levels being lousy and my diet not where it should be. I could feel that he was frustrated with me, but as a woman in my early forties I had lots of issues that didn't relate to diabetes. It got to the point that if something was wrong, I didn't even want to go to the doctor because I would always end up in the diabetes conversation and feel bad about myself."

"I tend to set high expectations for myself and for my patients." David said. "And I'm hard on myself when things don't go right. She was clearly very intelligent and hardworking. What could I be doing better?"

———

"Noncompliance" is a hot-button issue in medicine. Defined literally, it means the patient is not following the doctor's recommendations—whether for taking medications, showing up for an appointment, getting a test, or eating appropriately. In this model, Tracey would clearly be labeled noncompliant. However, the term has started to fall out of favor because of the paternalistic overtone and the implication that the patient is doing something bad. Now the term is "adherence," with the more neutral determination of whether a patient is able to adhere to an agreed-upon medical plan. As Tracey's story illustrates, adhering to a medical plan can be extremely difficult, with factors much more complex and multifaceted than a patient simply choosing not to do the right thing.

Heidi E. Hamilton, a linguistics researcher at Georgetown University, has been interested in the issue of nonadherence in diabetes because of its vast cost in both dollars and health. She wondered how communication issues might play a role in adherence to diabetes regimens.[1] Hamilton examined videotapes of twenty-four routine visits of patients with diabetes, plus individual interviews with the doctors and with the patients after the visits. In the office visits, the communication challenges were easy to see. The doctors tried all sorts of strategies to get their patients to adhere. At the most basic, there was the standard recitation of the facts and figures about diabetes. Then there were doctors who added more persuasion and emotion to this education effort, almost trying to sell their patients on the benefits of adherence. Some doctors nagged and harangued their patients. Others used scare tactics, trotting out the awaiting horrors of dialysis, blindness, amputations, impotence, and heart attacks. At the extreme end was the occasional doctor who implied that the patients might need to find another doctor if they didn't shape up soon. But as most doctors and most patients know (and any parent knows!), the strategy of repetitively hammering in the facts rarely achieves the desired outcome. Yet doctors seem to do it over and over again, despite the lack of results.

The first question to ask is why is adhering to a medical plan so arduous? Various studies suggest that 50–75 percent of patients have difficulty with adherence.[2] The answers were right there, Hamilton saw, plain as day—but only in the post-visit interviews. In these open-ended discussions, without the doctor present, patients spoke more forthrightly about what was happening in the trenches of real life. They knew *exactly* where the pitfalls and stumbling blocks lay.

Whether it was the cost of healthy food, the discomfort of insulin shots, the side effects of medications, the social pressures of eating, their complicated work schedules, the embarrassment of taking medications, the shame surrounding body image, the expense of glucometer supplies, the emotional eating to relieve anxiety, the cutting of pills in half to make an expensive prescription last longer, the conflicts with other family members, the simple longings for the foods of their youth—the patients knew precisely what the sources of nonadherence were. (Tellingly, not one patient cited lack of factual knowledge as the reason for not being able to adhere to a treatment plan.)

When Hamilton went back to the videos of the doctor-patient visits, none of this came up in conversation. Mainly the doctors spent their time trying to educate their patients, even though the post-visit interviews revealed that the patients knew all the relevant stats. "Patients are so varied as to what motivates and what challenges them," Hamilton told me. "They have so many issues in their lives that make diabetes hard to manage, but these issues don't come up in the regular doctor-patient encounter."

Research into adherence with blood pressure treatment by some of my colleagues at NYU reveals comparable findings.[3] When doctors dominate the conversation and focus on the strictly medical issues of the visit—as opposed to the psychosocial aspects—the risk of nonadherence to medications is three-fold higher. When patients are experiencing particularly stressful life situations such as inadequate housing or unemployment, doctors' avoidance of these issues is associated with a six-fold higher risk of nonadherence to medication. It's often hard for doctors to comprehend that there's much more to adherence than a patient just opening a bottle and swallowing a pill.

There is clearly an asymmetry between the doctor and the patient—doctors endlessly reciting the facts of the disease and patients with a store of crucial information that never gets on the table. Of course, some asymmetries in the medical relationship are a given; it is the patient with the illness and the doctor with the medical background. But other asymmetries are created, with both doctor and patient having a hand in it.

As I mentioned earlier, it is the patient who usually takes the lead when the visit starts, as it is the patient who made the appointment and came to the doctor. But within minutes, or usually seconds, the doctor snags that lead, steering the conversation in a particular direction—especially in the narrowly biomedical visit that Debra Roter described. This is not always a bad thing—the doctor may be drilling down to figure out the cause of a patient's symptom—but nevertheless there is a clear shift in who is leading.[4] This may be why patients' insider information about nonadherence never comes to light: doctors are too busy leading to stop and ask, and patients may feel that they don't have the opportunity or legitimacy to put their knowledge out there.

"Doctors," Hamilton noted, "use the blunt instrument of reciting the facts. They have the laudable goal of educating the patient but it can come across as simply reading the riot act over and over again."

David Baron was earnestly working to engage Tracey Pratt in caring for her diabetes. He used the tools he knew best: education and counseling. He also invested personal effort and caring to try to help Tracey understand the disease better. But for Tracey, it felt like getting the riot act read to her, over and over again, even though she knew that he meant well.

Tracey found herself avoiding the clinic more and more because every time she went she ended up feeling lousy about herself. "When I did have to go," she admitted with a guilty smile, "I would try to see the nurse practitioner instead of Dr. Baron. But Dr. B would always seem to find me! I would feel like 'He got me—now I'll have to hear it.' In retrospect I know that it was because he really cared but at the time it was like getting caught with your hand in the cookie jar."

"At some point," David said, "she'd flash that nice bright smile and tell me what I wanted to hear." He gave a self-deprecating laugh. "I'd fall for it every time. . . ."

It's very easy, especially in a busy clinic, for a patient who misses a few appointments to get lost in the shuffle. The more time that passes, the more easily he or she can fall through the cracks. But

David knew all too well that getting lost in the shuffle with un-controlled diabetes could have dreadful medical consequences, so he redoubled his efforts. "Even though she was trying to avoid visits with me," he said, "I kept looking for little ways to connect, hoping to nudge her back on track. I also wanted to show her my support and concern. So I was really surprised to learn, later on, that what I thought was support and concern, she perceived as overbearing."

"I remember one of our last visits before my one-year hiatus from the clinic," Tracey said. "I had come in for something completely unrelated and he brought the conversation back to diabetes again. He was frustrated with me and I was just as frustrated with him. That's when I started to avoid him. To get refills, I'd go to the pharmacy and ask *them* to call the clinic for refills. Anything to avoid seeing him in the clinic."

"Here was a patient who could really understand the medical is-sues," David said, "but it wasn't working out. It was hard for me not to take it personally."

"Things were getting worse," Tracey acknowledged, "but I was getting the message that it was because I wasn't doing the things I needed to be doing." The guilt and blame were more than she could handle, so she finally decided that she needed to switch doctors. Thinking it might be awkward to see a different doctor at the same clinic, she decided to go the whole hog and switch insurance plans and start at a different location.

"But it never happened," Tracey said, taking a self-mocking jab at herself, "because I missed the open enrollment to change insurance. In my heart of hearts, though, I knew that I wasn't doing what I needed to do to care for myself. I was mostly taking my medications but I wasn't as organized as I needed to be. Overall, I'm a type B person, which works well for teaching. But for diabetes you need to be type A."

On a Friday evening in December, Tracey stopped at the Lotus Café for a spicy tuna roll. The next morning she awoke with a stom-achache. Her friend Stanley had warned her about eating sushi from a place that used to be a Kentucky Fried Chicken and now she was paying the price. Either that or it was a stomach bug she'd caught from one of her students. Whatever it was, she didn't think much of it. She didn't call her doctor because it had been about a year now that she hadn't had much contact with the clinic.

In any case, she was too busy. She'd enrolled in a principal-certification program and had a paper due that week. Over the next few days she had worsening stomach cramps and then started vomiting. "I still thought it was a bug that would pass," she said, so didn't bother seeking medical attention. She ventured out to the Stop & Shop on Tuesday evening to buy some soup because she couldn't hold down any solid food. It was a chilly night with slippery black ice on the sidewalks. She inched her way to the store and promptly vomited in the restroom. On the way back, it was so cold that she could hardly draw a breath. She had to sit down on the icy front steps of her building because she couldn't muster the energy to turn the key in the door.

Once again, it was her practical mother who stepped in. Over the phone, Tracey's mother insisted that she go to the hospital. "I was still mainly concerned with getting this paper done that was due on Thursday," Tracey said, "but I was too weak to argue with her." Tracey was so short of breath that it was a struggle just to dial 911.

Tracey arrived in the emergency room semiconscious, severely dehydrated, with sky-high blood glucose and rock-bottom blood pressure. The pH level in her blood had plunged into acidic levels, near the range where the heart cells could be destabilized into cardiac arrest. "When they told me I would be admitted to the intensive-care unit," she recalled, "I realized that it was serious."

Even though Tracey Pratt had type 2 diabetes, she was in the throes of diabetic ketoacidosis (DKA), a life-threatening complication usually seen only in type 1 diabetes. The autoimmune process that underlies type 1 diabetes completely snuffs out the pancreas's ability to make insulin, so if a patient runs out of her insulin prescription, she can easily end up in the extreme situation of DKA. Patients with type 2 diabetes, by contrast, are still able to produce insulin. Though their bodies don't use that insulin effectively, the presence of a baseline amount usually protects them from DKA. So Tracey's descent into DKA was as unexpected as it was grim.

She was rushed to the ICU as liters of fluid were pumped into her veins to bolster her blood pressure. A round-the-clock insulin drip was initiated to ease down her glucose in a controlled manner. The electrolyte chaos in her blood was corrected, though gingerly—in DKA it's all too easy to slam the physiologic ballast in the other direction.

Tracey vaguely remembers seeing David in the emergency room, and even though she'd been irritated by him, it was still a comfort to see a familiar face amid the chaos. "You are very sick," she remembers him telling her, "but you will be okay." The reassurance was very meaningful to her, though most of that day was a blur. It took several days of intensive treatment for Tracey's metabolism to edge back from the brink.

It seemed that Tracey might have had a more severe type of diabetes than either she or David had suspected in the beginning. Certainly ending up in the ICU with DKA is not typical of patients with type 2 diabetes, though it is known to happen on occasion. Mixed in with the scare of this life-threatening episode was an odd element of relief for both David and Tracey. It wasn't that he was an ineffective doctor or that she was a "noncompliant" patient, but that they were dealing with a complicated and forceful illness thrust into their lives, one that was much thornier than either had expected. Tracey was bright and hardworking, struggling to fit an absolutely unwanted challenge into her already more-than-full life. David was well known as a compassionate and thoughtful doctor, dedicated to going the extra mile for his patients. Despite their efforts—as well as their missteps—the disease was a relentless challenge. Nevertheless, both doctor and patient realized that at some point they would have to talk about what had transpired between them over the past year or two.

"He tried to have that conversation with me every day in the ICU," Tracey recalled, "but I wasn't ready for it. But I didn't have the wherewithal to tell him that."

David remembers the tension. "She was reserved," he said, "only reluctantly engaging with me."

"The conversation was always about *me*," Tracey said. "Like, why I hadn't been to the clinic this past year. Honestly, it seemed more about his ego as a doctor than about me as a patient." For some doctors, there might be the temptation to say—or imply—"I told you so. If you had just done what you were supposed to do, none of this would have happened." But that isn't David's modus operandi. Mainly, he felt sad about the suffering Tracey had to endure, the miserable days in the ICU. When he had volunteered in the Dominican Republic those many years ago, he'd been stymied by his lack of skills. He'd been so frustrated to sit, impotent, on the sidelines while that man in the street experienced a seizure. "Now I have all this expertise that I didn't have in the DR," he reflected, his tone tinged with regret, "but I still can't always help my patients." But he also recognized that the ICU crisis might be a turning point for Tracey. She might now be able to trust him more and allow him to work with her more on her illness. She might now be able to focus more strongly on what she needed to do to take care of herself.

"My initial response to him," Tracey said, "was, 'I don't want you as my doctor. I want to change doctors.' He replied, 'If that's what you want, that's fine. I just want you to be okay.' I know he was trying to be nice but I don't think he picked up on how upset I was." When Tracey and I spoke about this, more than a year and a half after the event, she choked up while retelling the story. She was amazed that the illness and the confrontation were still so emotionally laden for her.

However, when the hospital discharge papers gave Tracey a follow-up appointment with David, she didn't object. "By the time I recovered from the DKA," she said, "I felt much better, so I felt okay about having an appointment with Dr. B. Despite my frustration I was still really glad he was my doctor."

At that first visit David readily acknowledged the situation. He opened with "I know you said you wanted another doctor . . ."

But Tracey's trademark pragmatism sailed right in. "It's all right," she said. "Let's just get on with it." She never viewed the situation as anyone's fault, so there didn't need to be any apology or forgiveness—on either side. And inside she was thinking, "Of all the doctors out there, I'd rather be in the care of someone who knows me than someone who doesn't."

David had been thinking about the ways he could best help Tracey in this next chapter of her medical care. The clinic had recently created a program for diabetes that involved shared medical appointments. A group of patients, all with diabetes, would come to the clinic at the same time. There would be nurses, nutritionists, podiatrists, pharmacists, and doctors all involved. Much of the visit, though, was patients helping other patients with the ins and outs of diabetes. David would still be her primary doctor, but there would now be an adjunctive team to offer extra support.

Tracey was hesitant at first but eventually gave it a try. It turned out to be an excellent fit, and very quickly Tracey became a leader in the group, the experienced voice who offered guidance to other patients. The multidisciplinary approach suited her busy schedule, as she was able to interface with many specialists at once. And the fact that the appointments were in the evenings meant her school schedule wouldn't be disrupted.

This also turned out to be an excellent fit for David and Tracey's doctor-patient relationship. Diabetes no longer had to dominate their visits, as there was now a whole team working on the disease. David and Tracey were able to focus on other aspects of Tracey's health that had been neglected by the overbearing shadow of the diabetes. The medical issues—diabetes and otherwise—improved markedly.

One year after this episode Tracey and David did something that was both very unusual and very brave. They sat together and told their stories in public. They spoke in front of an audience of patients, doctors, nurses, and medical staff as part of the Health Story Collaborative. Founded by Annie Brewster, an internist at Massachusetts General Hospital, the Health Story Collaborative encourages patients to tell their stories. During her medical training Brewster was diagnosed with multiple sclerosis and found herself seeking the stories of other patients to help her come to terms with the disease. Working with psychologist Jonathan Adler, Brewster has spent the past few years recording stories of patients with different illnesses and also helping them tell their stories publicly before audiences of family and friends.

The act of telling the story turns out to be very therapeutic for the teller, and hearing it is therapeutic for the listener.[5]

Brewster and Adler wondered what it might be like to have patients and their doctors tell their stories together. Tracey and David were the first pair in this experiment.[6] In front of the audience, they each spoke for twenty minutes, discussing their personal histories. David recounted picking corn as a child in Ohio, his experiences as a volunteer in the Dominican Republic. Tracey spoke about being a teacher and her drive to start a new life in Cambridge. And they each told the story of the illness that catapulted them—two random strangers, really—into intimate contact. They spoke frankly about how it was to work with the other person, and how difficult some of the moments were. Afterward, the moderator asked questions that encouraged a dialogue between them.

When I watched the video of this presentation, I was fascinated. It was intriguing to hear them each tell the tale—almost like having two movie cameras, placed at two different vantage points, shooting the same scene. You could pick out the factual trajectory of the diabetes and could also understand how each camera viewed the events differently. But the most interesting thing was that both views were realistic and accurate portrayals. There wasn't the stereotype of the noncompliant patient or the paternalistic doctor. As with Morgan Amanda and Juliet, there were two equally valid and plausible stories. Two equally objective accounts of the same set of facts.

What impressed me even more was how David and Tracey talked directly to each other about their experiences together, confronting their misunderstood efforts and communication mishaps. This was the first time I'd seen such an exchange. Doctors certainly talk to colleagues about their patients, and patients definitely talk to friends and family about their doctors. But it is almost unheard of to have doctors and patients talk directly to each other about their working relationship.

When I think about this, I realize that there's no real place in the medical world for this sort of communication, except perhaps in psychoanalysis, where issues of transference can be discussed. In regular medical encounters, the boundaries of doctor roles and patient roles prevent such conversation about the relationship and the communication.

Brewster and Adler acknowledge that "professional boundaries are certainly important."[7] But, they also note that "this obsession with boundaries has conspired with the pressures of efficiency . . . to remove some very personal (and important) elements of the patient-provider relationship."

What David and Tracey did was quite unusual. David admitted that it was challenging, but also noted that there was a "liberating feeling that we are all just people talking together." There was some awkwardness, of course. The audience was filled with his patients, fellow doctors, his staff, medical students, even his wife—all of whom know him and work with him in different ways. Nevertheless, it had a profound impact on him as a physician.

"I have a much better sense of Tracey's life and all the challenges that a chronic disease like diabetes has on one's life," David observed. "So it is easier to see her as a partner rather than me being the sole 'expert' and doling out advice. I must say, the former is much more satisfying."

For Tracey, it occurred to her how much she and David had in common with respect to their professional lives: "We both have jobs that serve the general public. We both spend an inordinate amount of time thinking about how to have the greatest impact on those we serve. Both of our jobs are often thankless; but I imagine that, like me, Dr. Baron knows that all the time and energy spent is well worth it when he has a positive impact on those he serves."

Diabetes has become a very matter-of-fact part of Tracey's life. It's not something she necessarily discloses to everyone, but neither is it something she hides. As is often instinctive in teachers, everything can be teaching material, and diabetes is no exception. She is a leader in the patient groups at the Cambridge Health Alliance but also uses diabetes in teaching her middle school students. Diabetes is a pillar of her life but it doesn't define her life.

"Some of the most positive moments in my life," Tracey later told me, "have occurred *since* being diagnosed with diabetes." In the relatively short span of time that diabetes has been in her life, Tracey has visited the Elmina slave castle in Ghana, climbed the Great Wall of China, learned how to merengue on a Havana rooftop, purchased her own home, returned to school, and completed a yearlong intensive program for a certificate of advanced graduate study in education administration.

And that's only what she's accomplished in her spare time. . . .

CHAPTER 6

What Works

You go to the doctor with a problem; the doctor prescribes a treatment. You, of course, hope it works. You hope your doctor has some evidence behind the treatment that she is offering you. We expect our doctors to practice evidence-based medicine, to make decisions based on good-quality research. We expect that they choose the blood pressure medications, chemotherapies, and cardiac treatments that offer the best-proven outcomes.

But what about how doctors speak? Is there evidence that the medical conversation influences clinical outcomes? On the surface, it seems hard to imagine that the words we doctors say to our patients, and how we say them, can have a potency comparable to the medications we prescribe, but a surprisingly robust body of research supports this. Given that words are a lot cheaper than medications—and rarely make you gain weight or break out in hives—this seems like a worthy avenue of exploration.

One of the earliest studies that showed a demonstrable effect of the simple act of talking was conducted in 1964.[1] As anyone who's undergone abdominal surgery knows, one of the worst hardships after surgery is pain. Postoperative pain, especially in the abdomen, is miserable and can require prodigious doses of narcotics to effectively control it. But narcotics produce a myriad of side effects ranging from nausea, vomiting, and itching to mental changes, drowsiness, and full respiratory arrest. For many patients—and their doctors—the intractable constipation can be the biggest torment. Thus, minimizing post-op narcotic use is a high priority for everyone on the medical playing field.

In the 1964 study, a group of about one hundred patients undergoing abdominal surgery was studied. The night before the operation, an anesthetist visited each patient to explain the surgery and anesthesia. For half the patients—randomly selected—the anesthetists added in a twenty-minute discussion about post-op pain. Patients were told that pain was a normal part of the process and that it was caused by muscle spasms. They were told where the pain would likely be located, when to expect it, and how long it would last. The anesthetist offered suggestions on how to relax the muscles to minimize the pain. Lastly, the anesthetists gave instructions on how to request pain medications if the relaxation techniques didn't work. The anesthetists were instructed to be enthusiastic in their presentation and express confidence that the pain would be relieved.

The control group did not receive this extra discussion. The surgeons who operated and took care of the patients after surgery had no idea who was in which group.

Looking back at this study from today, it doesn't seem surprising that the group with the extra discussion experienced less pain. Giving patients the information that they need—not necessarily the standard of care in 1964—goes a long way toward relieving the anxiety and fear that worsen pain. But what was impressive was the magnitude of the effect. The group with the extra discussion needed *half* the amount of pain medication that the control group needed. When it comes to serious medications like narcotics, a reduction by half is a remarkable improvement in medical care.

But the real shocker was that these patients were discharged from the hospital three days earlier than those in the control group! A typical day in the hospital now costs upward of four thousand dollars,[2] so here is a decidedly low-tech intervention—a twenty-minute conversation—that saved more than twelve thousand dollars in present-day money, and spared patients many days of pain and misery. (And as an internist, I will add that any intervention that minimizes constipation is worthy of a gold medal in and of itself.)

This landmark study ignited the field, as researchers began investigating in earnest to see if and how doctors' communication could have effects on patients' health comparable to standard medical interventions. One study that caught my eye focused on back pain. Low back pain is as common as oxygen. If there has been a single day in my practice that back pain has *not* come up, I certainly can't recall it. Once the serious but exceedingly rare causes of back pain have been eliminated—cancer, infection—and the diagnosis is regular old muscular back pain, physical therapy is the treatment of choice. When I send my patients for physical therapy, I think of it in terms of the exercises that the patients will be guided to do, sometimes accompanied by other modalities such as ultrasound, massage, and mild electrical stimulation.

What I don't typically think of is how the communication between the therapist and my patient will affect the pain. A group of Canadian researchers divided 120 patients with back pain into four groups.[3] Half the patients received the electrical stimulation and half received sham stimulation (all the equipment is set up, but the electrical current is never activated). Because electrical stimulation causes a mild pins-and-needle sensation, the patients in the sham group were told that the machine was on but that with this "new machine" they might not feel any tingling at all.

As had been shown in many other studies, sham treatment (i.e., placebo) works quite well: these patients had a 25 percent reduction in their levels of pain. This by itself is impressive. Those patients who got the real stimulation did better, though; their pain levels decreased by 45 percent, so we know that the electrical stimulation actually does something.

Each of these two groups, however, was further divided in half. One half experienced limited conversation from the physical therapist. The therapist briefly explained the procedure but then told the patient that everything needed to be quiet during the treatment. With the other half, the therapists engaged in conversation the entire time. The therapists were striving to create a "therapeutic alliance" with the patients in this group and so asked open-ended questions, listened attentively, and inquired about how the back pain was affecting the patients' lives. The therapists expressed empathy about the patients' situation but also offered words of encouragement and optimism about getting better. There was plenty of eye contact and touch.

Unsurprisingly, the patients who had the more engaged therapists did better, but it's the degree of improvement that's impressive. Patients who underwent sham treatment—no electrical stimulation—but had therapists who actively communicated with them reported a 55 percent decrease in their pain. Think about that for a minute: the communication with the physical therapist was *more effective* than the treatment by itself (a 55 percent reduction in pain with communication alone as opposed to a 45 percent reduction in pain with just electrical treatment).

The patients who had the electrical stimulation accompanied by the engaged physical therapists were the clear winners, with a 77 percent reduction in pain. This type of study provides hard evidence for what healers, shamans, witch doctors, and assorted mystics have known for millennia: that a substantial portion of "healing" comes from the personal connection that is formed with the patient. It's no great secret, of course. Wise physicians and experienced nurses (not to mention astute patients) have also keyed into this, even if only subconsciously. Nevertheless, it's intriguing to see this effect borne out in controlled scientific studies.

These studies bring me to the whole idea of placebo. The placebo effect, as most people know, is a change in someone's health from a treatment that contains no active medical substance. The effect is well known, which is why every clinical trial worth its salt is placebo-controlled. The treatment under investigation must be compared with a placebo, not to "doing nothing," because the placebo group always registers an effect. The treatment has to score better than placebo, otherwise it's deemed useless.

But outside of research, placebo has been viewed with suspicion. Using placebos in actual clinical medicine is considered shady, if not downright unethical. But communication plays an enormous role in placebo and the eschewal of using placebo in treatment is starting to ease. I had occasion to employ a placebo one night during my second year of medical residency, though even to this day I'm not sure whether I did the right thing.

It was well past midnight on the AIDS ward at Bellevue Hospital in New York City, at a time when this ward was overflowing with patients. Despite the late hour, the nurses and doctors were still rushing about at full speed, as the admissions continued to surge in, each more feverish and emaciated than the previous. But even the AIDS ward eventually quieted down for the night. Except, that is, for the howler.

The howler was a patient in his thirties who'd earned his nickname for his nightly bouts of wailing. He was already receiving hefty doses of pain medication, yet he kept screaming to the nurses about his pain. This went on, night after night, despite extensive medical evaluations to see if there were any missed explanations for his pain.

Nothing seemed to help and the nightly yowling was agitating the other patients, not to mention driving the nursing staff to distraction. (We doctors had patients on many wards so were constantly in and out of the ward. The nurses, on the other hand, were staffed to a specific ward and so could not escape the howler.) The head nurse stat-paged me at 3 a.m. "You have to *do* something," she said, her voice boiling with apoplexy, "before somebody marches in there and strangles him."

Reluctantly, I trudged back to the patient's room. I'd been on my feet for more hours than I could count and this was my fourth visit to the howler that night. By this point, we were both pretty exasperated with each other. He was sullen and cranky; I was exhausted and at my wits' end. I watched the patient writhing in bed and felt bad for him, but his moans burrowed into my brain, deflating my last three functioning neurons. The room was stuffy from that medicalized staleness that only hospitals can brew up. Would this night ever end?

I rummaged around in my pockets to see what I could come up with and pulled out a vial of saline. On a whim, I plucked a syringe from another pocket and slowly peeled back the wrapper. Stepping in closer to the patient's bedside, I cocked back the syringe and drew up 1 cc of the plain saline. "You know about Tylenol, right?" I said to the patient, who was continuing to twist within his bed sheets. "And you've heard of Tylenol number three, the kind with codeine."

I leaned forward and held up the liquid-filled syringe close to the patient's face. "There's even a Tylenol number four." I slowly removed the cover off the needle and it glistened in the fluorescent lights. "But *this*"—and here I paused for dramatic effect—"*this* is Tylenol number *five!*"

The patient stopped howling and gave me an interested look. Without a word he lowered his pajamas and allowed me to inject the saline into his gluteus maximus. I disposed of the syringe in the nearby sharps box and then pulled up a chair to his bedside. The patient and I waited together, allowing the minutes to tick unhurriedly by.

After what seemed like a mutually agreeable time, I stood up and bid him good night. The patient put his head to the pillow and promptly fell asleep. The ward was silent for the rest of the night.

I did feel guilty that I had committed an outright deception with this patient—something I knew was a true no-no. On the other hand, it was the first time he got a full night of sleep, to say nothing of all the other patients on the ward and the rest of the staff. (The head nurse bought me coffee and a bagel the next morning and we remained buddies for all the years of my residency.)

When I related this story to Ted J. Kaptchuk, director of the program in placebo studies at Harvard Medical School, he gave a sigh of recognition. "We all have our moments of desperation," he said drily. "Usually around midnight."

Kaptchuk does not condone deception, but research bears out that *how* caregivers present and administer treatments has a powerful effect on clinical outcomes. In an ingenious Italian study, patients who'd just undergone chest surgery were all given the appropriate doses of narcotics for their post-op pain.[4] For patients in one group, the narcotics were automatically administered in their IVs. The patients had been told in advance that IV pain meds would be given reliably over the course of the day but they were not given any indication at the time each dose began. Nor were any doctors or nurses present when the medication began to drip in. For the patients in the other group the medication was given on the same schedule but a doctor injected it manually.

The patients in the latter group consistently achieved more main relief than the patients who received the medicine unknowingly in their IVs, even though it was the same dose of medication given at the same intervals. The rituals the doctors performed—coming to the bedside, acknowledging the patients' pain, drawing up the medication, visibly injecting it into the IV, and discussing the expected benefits, not to mention the attention and caring that comes with the presence of an actual human being—effected as much pain relief as *doubling* the dose of the medication.

Kaptchuk describes placebo not as the traditional sugar pill but as "everything that surrounds a medical treatment": how caregivers describe the medication, how they administer it, the expectations they offer for the medicine, their tone of voice, their words of connection, their strength of eye contact. In short, everything that doctors and nurses do in an interaction with a patient.

As I mentioned, healers and shamans have known intuitively about the importance of this interaction since the dawn of time. Before we had treatments that could actually impact the pathology of disease—antibiotics, chemotherapy, stents, organ transplants, transfusions—the "everything else" was the mainstay of medical care, and in many cases it was remarkably effective.

But in the twentieth century, now that there were actual medical treatments, placebos were considered psychological mumbo jumbo, more akin to hypnotism than real medicine. The biological breakthrough came in 1978, when researchers showed that not only was the placebo effect real, but that it could be reversed by administering naloxone—a chemical that blocks our endorphins.[5] Endorphins are intriguing neurochemicals that act as our homegrown painkillers. The term, in fact, was coined by my PhD adviser Eric Simon as a contraction of "endogenous morphine" because that's how these neurochemicals behaved, just like morphine.[6] (I spent several wonderful years escaping med school in Eric's lab, as we researched the biochemistry of the receptors for these endorphins.)

Despite this biological underpinning, doctors and nurses still feel uneasy when it comes to placebos. Somehow administering them seems wrong, unethical, deceptive. But patients, it turns out, are more flexible in their thinking. Kaptchuk has demonstrated that patients experience symptom relief even when they are told quite plainly that they are getting a placebo.In one of his experiments, patients with irritable bowel syndrome randomly received either a placebo or no treatment at all.[7] The patients in the placebo group were explicitly told that the pills were made of inert substances. They were also told that research had demonstrated that placebos relieve pain.

This "open-label" placebo is a direct contrast to standard clinical trials in which participants don't know if they are getting the active medication or the placebo. The blinding in clinical trials is deliberate because, presumably, if you *knew* you were getting the blank pills you wouldn't experience any placebo effect and the true effect of the test medication couldn't be accurately teased out.

In Kaptchuk's study, however, the patients knowingly took the placebo. There was no effort to dress it up with the chance that they might be receiving an active medication. Yet after three weeks these patients who openly took an inert pill experienced a decrease in their symptoms and an increase in their quality-of-life ratings. In this study, and in other surveys that Kaptchuk has done, patients can be quite amenable to open-label placebos.[8] As one of my patients once told me, "If it gets rid of the pain, I don't care if it's a dill pickle!" Anyone who has struggled with chronic pain would be likely to agree.

The ethics are evolving but the general consensus is that transparency is the bottom line. What I did as a young and desperate resident wouldn't pass muster because I had deceived my patient about the medication. But if I'd told him honestly that it was inert saline and if he'd given informed consent, it could have been a reasonable treatment option. From what Kaptchuk has found in his studies, my patient still might have experienced relief even knowing I was injecting him with nothing but saline, especially if we had been able to have a compassionate conversation about his pain. Relieving suffering (without causing more harm), after all, is what the Hippocratic oath is all about.

I've found myself utilizing some aspects of placebo medicine in my clinical practice. It comes up most often in patients with vague pain and fatigue, for whom the medical workup has not revealed a specific cause. Many of these patients have additional psychological and social stresses that compound their situations. Frequently they will ask if a multivitamin will give them more energy. In the past I would say no because there are no scientific studies to demonstrate this, and also because in the absence of a vitamin deficiency there's not much for a basic multivitamin pill to do. Now, however, I take a different approach. I will say something along the lines of "Many of my patients find that they have more energy when they take a multivitamin." I'm not lying, because many of my patients have indeed said so. I'll be honest with them that we don't have rigorous scientific data, but I'll also point out that research studies deal with average effects over populations; they can't predict how an individual person might respond.

I would never, of course, say this regarding a medication with a more toxic side-effect profile, but given that there's little downside to an inexpensive multivitamin I'll encourage them to give it a try and offer them my optimistic take that it's definitely possible they'll feel better. If it helps, we've accomplished something. If not, we're no worse than before. Most of my patients still have symptoms but there are always a few patients who come back at the next visit and swear they feel much better on the vitamin pill. There are some who argue that it is unethical to promote placebo-type medications to patients. But increasingly, many say it would be unethical *not* to give placebo a try in situations where patients are not getting relief from traditional means (and where it would not cause harm or otherwise replace a necessary treatment).

Kaptchuk views placebo as just one of the many things in the tool kit of medicine. It would never be a substitute for appropriate medical care but it is something that can enhance medical care greatly. Wise doctors and nurses already know this. They've found, usually just by personal experience, that their "everything else"—respect, attention, comfort, empathy, communication, touch—often forms the lion's share of medical care, no deception required.

A key part of the "everything else" of placebo is clearly the communication between doctor and patient. One salutary thing communication can do is reduce anxiety, which in turn can reduce pain. A thirty-eight-year-old woman came to my office with concerns about chest pain. She was worried—as most people with chest pain are—that it could be a heart condition. We spoke about her symptom and she told me it occurred twice a month and lasted for thirty minutes at a time. It wasn't precipitated by exertion—in fact, she had a physically strenuous job in a warehouse transporting heavy boxes. She regularly climbed several flights of stairs during a typical workday. I also learned that she was under a lot of stress because recently her hours had been cut back and her economic situation was now in jeopardy. The stress was agitating her sleep but she was trying to keep everything under wraps so as not to upset her older mother, whom she lived with and supported financially.

The chest pain she described was a long distance from classic angina—pressing chest pain brought on reliably by exertion, relieved by rest, lasting only several minutes. Her robust daily physical activity was the equivalent of a cardiac stress test that indicated a heart with plenty of oxygen and blood supply. As a premenopausal woman of thirty-eight, her statistical risk for heart disease was quite low. Plus she had an alternative explanation—life stress—not to mention a normal physical exam and EKG. So by the end of our conversation, without injecting any delay by ordering additional tests, I was able to tell her that I was entirely convinced this pain was not from her heart, that her heart was extremely healthy.

Her relief was palpable—she sat back in her chair with a long sigh and an even wider smile. Apparently she'd spent the past few months nursing a growing conviction that her heart was failing and that she might no longer be able to do her job or care for her mother. At our next visit a few months later, she said that her chest pain had simmered down, and though it was still there, she hardly noticed it.

Maybe she'd been having muscular soreness in her chest from her heavy lifting and it had improved on its own. But maybe my reassurance that her heart was not compromised offered a placebo effect.

Maybe it allowed her to relax enough to stop tensing the muscles that might have been contributing to her pain.

Reassurance that you are not in imminent danger, just by itself, can go a long way toward easing pain. Even for patients who *are* in imminent danger—those with terminal illness, for example—reassurance that they will not be alone in their illness, that their comfort and dignity will be attended to, that their advance directives will be honored, that their passage to death will be eased as much as possible—offers tremendous comfort and diminution of pain.

Reassurance may act physiologically by decreasing cortisol and adrenaline and perhaps increasing endorphins, which might directly reduce the neural perception of pain. Or reassurance may act cognitively by shifting the focus of concern so that the pain is no longer front and center. Either way, reassurance is a crucial part of the "everything else" that doctors and nurses do that decreases pain and discomfort.

A second way communication might offer placebo effect is by raising expectations. When I tell a patient, "Many of my patients have found that they have more energy when they take a multivitamin," I'm raising expectations. When Ted Kaptchuk told his ulcerative colitis subjects that the placebo they were taking had been shown in clinical trials to decrease pain, he was raising expectations. Now you could make the argument that this is a bit of huckstering, but in fact there is a good deal of evidence that expectation can affect the biology of pain perception.

In an intriguing study on pain perception,[9] twenty-two healthy volunteers were given a painful stimulus (a hot pad placed on the calf) and also an intravenous narcotic (similar to morphine) to relieve the pain. At the same time, their heads were conveniently positioned in an fMRI (functional MRI) machine, so researchers could document which parts of their brains were activated during the study.

The participants went through four rounds of the experiment. Each round was identical—the hot pad was placed on the calf and then the pain medication was infused into the IV—and the patients had to rank how much pain they felt. In the first round inert saline (placebo) rather than the actual medication was infused into the IV. This established a baseline pain score.

In the second round the pain medication was administered silently, without the patient being told. The medication clearly worked because the pain scores were lower, even without the patients being explicitly informed that the medication was starting.

In the third round it was announced that the medication infusion "would be now started by the anesthetist." As you might guess, being told that the medicine was about to start rolling in raised expectations and enhanced the pain relief. In fact, just having this positive expectation *doubled* the relief.

In the fourth round researchers announced that "the infusion would be stopped" in order to investigate potential "rebound effects" (pain that worsens after medications are discontinued). The medication, however, was actually given, just as it had been in the earlier rounds. But the subjects now had negative expectations—not only that they were not getting any pain meds, but that the pain might actually worsen. The negative expectation indeed wiped out the effects that the positive expectation in the third round had offered. Not only that, it also wiped out any baseline effect of the medication (the pain relief in round two). In the end, the simple act of negative expectation blocked the *entire* biological effect of a potent intravenous narcotic.

This is a fascinating finding: our expectations can be as influential as an actual medication. Now you could argue that maybe the subjects gave the answers they thought the researchers wanted (more pain relief when the medication was given, less pain relief when the medication was supposedly turned off). But the fMRI readings offered tantalizing suggestions about a biological explanation. When the study subjects received the medication along with a positive expectation, there was an increase in activity of the brain areas known to be involved in pain relief (these areas, incidentally, light up regardless of whether pain relief is from a narcotic or from placebo). In contrast, when the pain medication was administered along with a negative expectation, there was reduced brain activity in these areas.

While these are only experimental data, they bolster the idea that how doctors and nurses frame a treatment can have profound effects on how patients experience the results of that treatment. Earlier in my career I made efforts to present treatment options as soberly as possible to my patients. I laid out the risks and benefits so the patient could make a reasoned decision. I still do that, of course, but now I also try to frame things as optimistically as possible, within reason. I don't want to be a Pollyanna or paint unrealistic expectations for treatments that offer little value. But if we've chosen a path of treatment together, I try to invest both of our expectations in the right direction. Our communications might be a bit of placebo, but if it can help without causing side effects then it seems like a legitimate medical intervention to pursue.

What about adherence? What parts of the doctor-patient communication contribute to—or detract from—adherence? As Tracey Pratt and the work of Heidi E. Hamilton demonstrated, nonadherence is rarely about indifference or ignorance on the part of the patient, though that's what doctors often assume. Rather, it's usually the realities of life that seem to conspire against a patient's efforts to fully adhere to a treatment plan. It's been estimated that patients are able to follow doctors' recommendations—for medications, tests, therapy, diet, consultations—only about half the time.[10] That leaves a substantial number of patients who are missing out on the potential benefits of these recommendations. Many things have been posited to improve adherence: nurse visits, social-work counseling, follow-up phone calls, electronic reminders, home delivery of medications, health coaches, economic incentives.

Improved communication is certainly one of those things, but the devil for all of these interventions is in the magnitude of effect. The medical system needs to know how much bang there is for the buck before it chooses where to invest resources. So a team of scientists examined more than fifty years of research,[11] using the technique of meta-analysis to combine the results of one hundred individual studies. (These studies encompassed a total of forty-five thousand patients.) If all of these data are taken together, patients of doctors with good communication skills are more than twice as likely to have good adherence to medical recommendations, compared with patients whose doctors had poor communication skills. That's a 100 percent improvement, for those of you who prefer percentages.

For a rough comparison to a medical intervention that's considered high value, the benefit of statins in preventing heart attacks in patients with atherosclerotic disease is about 33 percent: those who take statins are a third less likely to have a heart attack as those who don't. Improved communication is a remarkable medical intervention that can rank in the big leagues (and of course doesn't even reach the hem of statins when it comes to cost).

One thing often believed to improve doctor-patient connection is humanizing the experience. Doctors sometimes attempt to do this by bringing in their own humanity, presenting themselves as real people, and not just as a stock figure in a white coat. Allowing personal details to enter the communication between doctor and patient is a common occurrence—estimates suggest that physician self-disclosure occurs in up to a third of routine office visits.[12] But is this actually helpful for the patient?

A couple of years ago I had a new patient in her midthirties, Anita Lyons. I found the medical care of Anita Lyons overwhelming from the get-go. She weighed nearly three hundred pounds and her diabetes was raging out of control. She suffered from asthma but continued to smoke to ease her anxiety. Her obesity was severe enough to constrict her mobility, but the constant stress in her life led her to overeat.

Ms. Lyons had been raised in a family beset with psychiatric, medical, and social challenges, and now the cycle seemed to be replicating itself. Her three children all had emotional and educational needs that required intensive services.

She couldn't figure out how to get a handle on her life, and as her new physician, I wasn't sure how to get a handle on it, either. Should I work on her diabetes first? Her smoking? Her weight? Her asthma?

Her anxiety and stress? Her life seemed frighteningly out of control. On what, I wondered, could we connect?

In the middle of our first visit her cell phone rang. She glanced at the caller ID then looked apologetically toward me. "It's my son's teacher," she said. I told her to please take the call. As a parent of three school-age children, I well understood how hard it could be to reach a teacher and how critical such calls were.

"I know my son missed two assignments," Ms. Lyons said into the phone, as I scrolled through her labs. "Sometimes he's anxious after therapy sessions, so I have to give him time on the playground." She paused and listened to the teacher. "We keep a chart," she said, "and he gets a check mark for each homework he finishes."

As she carried on the conversation I found myself feeling more connected to her. I knew about the driving necessity of playground time. I knew about the charts and the checks required to keep children focused on their tasks. My kids were about the same age as hers and I was all too familiar with the frenetic juggling required to keep up with three children and their schedules and their laundry and their homework and their lunches and their tantrums. I also knew the awkward sensation of explaining details of a life to a teacher, feeling like your messy reality won't pass muster.

When she hung up the phone she apologized for the interruption. "Don't worry," I reassured her. "Teacher calls are important." I was about to continue, to offer her some of our commonalities, thinking that common ground could offer us a good start on a working relationship.

But then I stopped myself. A week earlier I'd had a visit with one of my long-term patients—a Polish woman in her sixties who has been alone, and lonely, for as long as I've known her. At the end of our visit, she asked why there weren't any new pictures of my children; the photo on my desk was more than three years old.

"I never get around to printing any photos," I said sheepishly. "They just sit on my phone." She then leaned toward the cell phone sitting on my desk, somewhat expectantly. I debated what to do. I wasn't sure if sharing a personal photo was okay, but I also didn't want to seem imperious or cut off her very human gesture. I figured it would be okay to show her one quick photo. After all, we'd known each other for so many years by this point. I quickly dug up a family photo from my phone.

My patient broke into a wistful smile when she saw the photo. "What a happy family you have," she said. "Your husband looks like such a nice person. Your kids look so smart." The plaintiveness in her voice was so palpable, and I suddenly realized what a mistake I'd made. I'd thought it would strengthen our bond to share a bit of my life. But it turned out it may have had the opposite effect, as she projected onto my life some of the things that were missing in hers.

I quickly closed the photo, embarrassed at the awkward dynamics. There likely were some patients for whom the addition of the human element of the doctor's life might be helpful, but this patient probably wasn't one of them. I felt that I might have done something detrimental.

And so as I sat with Ms. Lyons, a woman who in many ways was so vastly different from me, I wondered if sharing some of the commonalities we did have would enhance our alliance and give us a better chance at tackling her medical issues.

In the end I decided to keep quiet. I couldn't be sure if such disclosure would offer solidarity or inadvertently toss in a monkey wrench. Instead, I simply acknowledged how challenging the situation with her children must be. I offered my admiration for her efforts and pointed out her successes.

She reddened slightly but smiled. "Raising kids is harder than I'd ever imagined."

"I know," I said. I wanted to say that I really did know, but I decided to leave it at that.

Research has borne out that doctors' self-disclosures often turn out not to be as helpful in addressing patients' concerns or building rapport as doctors presume them to be.[13] The attempt to empathize is certainly genuine: "My father also had lung cancer; I know how difficult it can be" or "I also had knee surgery; I know how hard the recovery is." But patients sometimes interpret these as disruptive, as the focus is shifted off them onto the doctors. In primary-care visits these self-disclosures are associated with lower patient satisfaction.[14]

Patients of doctors who disclosed personal details gave lower ratings of both friendliness and reassurance.

Interestingly, the opposite effect was found with surgeons. In the same study it was shown that patients of surgeons who offered self-disclosures gave higher ratings of friendliness, reassurance, and overall satisfaction. This may be because surgical visits often revolve around a single procedure for which the anxiety level of the patient is high and also focused. Personal reassurances—"My father had a bypass and he did just fine"—may do a lot to reduce fear, even though the outcome of the surgeon's father has no actual bearing on how the patient will fare. Primary-care medical visits, on the other hand, typically cover many areas of the patients' medical conditions, with no specific event such as an operation to focus on. Doctors' disclosures may feel like unwelcome sidetracks in these scenarios.

The desire to share commonalities is a human impulse. I'm not suggesting that doctors should never do this. Rather, doctors need to think before they do so reflexively and ask themselves if these particular details will offer assistance or if they will instead detract from the singularity of the patient's experience. Most important, if the doctor is sharing some personal details, the conversation needs to be steered promptly back to the patient, where it properly belongs. In my experience, when my patient asks about my life, or I find myself considering sharing something personal, as with Ms. Lyons, I realize that it always comes from the desire to kindle empathy. Despite all the advances of technology, medicine is still fundamentally a human endeavor, and whenever two human beings attempt to connect, empathy is the key building block upon which a relationship is created.

Empathy is often thought of as an emotion or a feeling. It's classically defined as the ability to put yourself in someone else's shoes and to understand how that person is feeling. But empathy qualifies as a communication skill as well. For empathy to be effective in medicine, the doctor has to communicate that empathy to the patient.[15] The doctor could be the most emotionally sensitive hominoid on the planet, steeped in the patient's culture and life story, willing to donate a kidney, a lung, and both corneas to the patient if need be, but without the ability to communicate that empathy, it will be meaningless for the patient.

So can empathy—with its critical reliance on communication—affect patient outcomes? One seminal study examined nearly nine hundred patients and divided them into three groups, depending on whether their doctors scored low, medium, or high on a question-naire that measured empathy.[16] For those patients lucky enough to have doctors with high empathy scores, 56 percent had good diabetes control and 59 percent had good cholesterol control. Of patients with doctors who scored low on the empathy scale, only 40 percent had good diabetes control and 44 percent had good cholesterol control. Using statistical analysis to control for age, gender, and health insur-ance, the researchers found that empathy was a significant contribu-tor to the positive outcomes.

This, of course, is a study that measures an "association" between empathy and the positive outcomes. Despite statistical controls, there could be something else that caused the results. Maybe the low-empathy doctors had dismal hygiene and the resulting BO was too distracting for the patients to pay attention to their diabetes. Maybe the offices of the high-empathy doctors offered cloth gowns rather than paper gowns, so their patients weren't experiencing frost-bite and thus were better able to hear what the doctor was saying. You never know what the confounding factors might be . . .

Another group of researchers set out to test the effects of empathy with a slightly stronger study design that used randomization, in this case with the ordinary, annoying, common cold.[17] More than seven hundred patients were randomly placed into three groups as soon as they presented with cold symptoms. One group didn't even see a doctor. The second group had "usual care" with a doctor. The third group saw doctors who, like the engaged physical therapists in the study I mentioned earlier in the chapter, made a special effort to con-nect with the patients. They listened closely and specifically worked to empathize with the patients' situation. They were also optimistic about a good prognosis.

The researchers were most interested in the patients' perceptions of empathy, so they had the patients rate the doctors on empathy and communication skills. The doctors who scored the highest were mostly from the "enhanced visit" group, though a few were from the regular-care group.

Patients who were taken care of by this high-scoring group of doctors did better than the other patients. They had a 17 percent decrease in severity of their colds, compared with patients who saw the other doctors, and the duration of their colds was shorter (5.9 days versus 7 days). These may not seem like large numbers, but one day less with your nose dripping into your coffee and your head stuffed with cotton is a valuable benefit in my book.

The researchers speculated that there might be a cellular basis for these results, so they examined the levels of white blood cells and inflammatory markers (interleukin-8) present in the nasal mucosa. Both of these biological markers dropped more profoundly in those patients with high-scoring doctors compared with patients of the other doctors. Though it doesn't offer proof, this study hints at some biological mechanisms that may underlie the positive effects of good communication and connection. It's possible that levels of cortisol and adrenalin are lowered when good communication lowers anxiety levels.

However, most researchers in the field believe the effects are more indirect. Improving communication can help patients understand instructions better or feel more confident about their ability to manage their disease. This may make them more likely to fill their prescriptions and take their medications, or follow their doctors' advice to take the day off from work and just sleep for twenty-four hours. With more empathetic communication, patients might feel safe enough to confide uncomfortable information that they might have otherwise been too embarrassed to share—a hidden eating disorder, a genital symptom, financial constraints—allowing the doctors to tailor the treatment appropriately. Doctors who take the time to understand patients' family lives and living conditions might be able to prescribe a medication that is more affordable or enlist a family member to help out with medical care or offer a discreet way to obtain treatment for an embarrassing condition.

Patients who feel stigmatized during their medical encounters— because of obesity, for example, or mental illness or substance abuse or gender identity or their racial or ethnic group—are more likely to drop out of the medical system entirely. But with empathetic doctors who take more time to connect, these patients may stay engaged in medical care and get the treatment they need. These indirect patterns probably explain most of the successes seen in studies of communication in medicine.[18]

What's tantalizing is that it doesn't require much additional effort on the part of the physician to have a meaningful effect. Nearly every good-quality study that gave the physician a concrete step to take resulted in better communication and improved patient satisfaction. Whether it was getting doctors to ask more open-ended questions, or to elicit the patient's concerns, or to set a clear agenda, or to inquire about the patient's life beyond the illness, or to involve the patient when choosing a treatment plan, or just to express more empathy—nearly any attention paid to these skills easily improved communication.[19] Now, whenever you bring up these kinds of studies in medical circles, there's always a good dose of eye rolling. Even doctors who intuitively understand the importance of good communication and connection with patients get a little impatient when you start talking about the hokier-sounding soft stuff. It doesn't have the same satisfying heft as the multicenter clinical trials of cardiac stents with tens of thousands of patients in twenty different countries run by fifteen of the top academic medical centers, with budgets that rival the national GDPs of respectable midsize nations.

I sympathize with this because I, too, have a similar reaction. It doesn't feel like "real" medicine and the gut reaction of most doctors is to push it to the side, somewhere near the viper-fish broth that torpedoes heart attacks in mid-clot and the Paraguayan cactus powder that evaporates cellulite in three short weeks for only $49.95 plus tax. Even with scientific evidence, we doctors still find this squishy stuff hard to embrace.

When I try to dissect out why doctors are so leery, I come up with two reasons. One is that these less-tangible components of medicine—communication, connection, empathy—are harder to measure than glucose levels or numbers of strokes. Although research in these fields has progressed significantly in the past few decades, it still lags in size and depth compared with the mega-trials of oncology treatments and cardiovascular outcomes. Plus you can't really write a prescription for communication or empathy, so it doesn't feel as real as other medical treatments (and how on earth would you convince the insurance company that this constitutes actual medical care and should be reimbursed the same way that endoscopies are?).

But the second reason is, I think, the more profound one. Communication, empathy, and connection are not things doctors typically learn in medical school. Med schools are beginning to pay attention to these skills but they are usually seen as add-ons, curricularly dwarfed by pathology, biochemistry, surgery, cardiology, obstetrics, pediatrics, and the like. These straight-science fields are the solid purviews of doctors, whereas those softer skills, well, anyone could use them. And, in fact, many other practitioners do. Alternative healers of all stripes make heavy use of these skills, which explains the surging popularity of alternative medicine. It also explains much of their effectiveness: as the physical therapy study demonstrated, much pain can be relieved with just good communication, empathy, and connection.

Herein lies the rub: something that simple and intuitive, something that doesn't require specialized knowledge, can feel threatening to a physician who has spent a decade training to acquire unique medical knowledge (and $100,000 worth of student-loan debt). I mean, it's not a lot of sweat off anyone's back to be a more engaged communicator, and if it doubles your patient's pain relief—why not? It's the very simplicity, I think, the *lack* of sweat off one's back, that makes it seem so squishy and simplistic to we doctors who frame ourselves in the scientific mold. There's something vaguely discomfiting to realize that the techniques shamans used centuries ago can sometimes be as effective as our pharmaceuticals backed by million-dollar mega-trials.

How can we help doctors overcome their reflex hesitation and feel comfortable adopting some of these simple but effective techniques? I put this question to Richard Street, a professor of communications at Texas A&M University. He readily acknowledged the difficulty of getting buy-in from doctors, and so whenever he gives lectures to doctors, he presents his research within a strictly scientific frame-work, emphasizing rigorous research studies. But then he flipped the question back to me, knowing that I am an ever-struggling student of the cello. "To become a musician," he said, "you need to acquire all the technical skills, right? The notes, the chords, the scales. This is the *science* of music. But when you *play* music, especially when you improvise, this is the art of music."

When Street described the doctor-patient interaction as an im-prov, the metaphor really hit home. While I don't improvise on the cello—I'm still trying to get a handle on the stuff that's already been written, thank you very much—I'm in absolute awe of musicians who *can* improvise. As I've learned more about music, I've come to under-stand that improvisation is less about making it up on the spot and more about reaching into your bag of tools and putting these tools together in new and creative ways. There is, of course, plenty of off-the-cuff artistic inspiration, but improvisers are generally utilizing well-honed musical techniques. Astute listeners familiar with basic music theory can pick out these tools as they spontaneously erupt—arpeggios, inversions, diminished seventh scales, syncopation, theme and variation, classic riffs. We tend to think of this as the purview of jazz musicians in performance, but Bach, Mozart, and Stravinsky were improvising as well; they were just doing it on the page rather than on stage.

And so it is with doctors and patients. Some encounters are straightforward but many are unpredictable. "Each person," Street said, "is responding to the other person's moves." Both are impro-vising to a certain degree. The wise doctor—and the wise patient, as well—will reach into her bag of tools and extract what is most needed for that particular person at that particular time. Communi-cation techniques are an additional set of tools to add to the bag to render the selection bigger and ultimately more useful. Corine Jansen is one person who has been vigorously expanding that bag of tools, and from a bracingly low-tech perspective.

CHAPTER 7

Chief Listening Officer

To most of the world, Amsterdam is the paragon of orderliness. Tidy streets with well-mannered citizens on rule-abiding bicycles, quaint canals lined with well-behaved flowers in faultless color coordination, canvas-ready windmills, and well-tended verdant fields with just enough ruggedness to justify seven shades of Prussian green, palette knife, and wool beret cocked just so. Amid this Dutch orderliness, Corine Jansen grew up immersed in conflict. Her first contact with her mother's mental illness was when she was seven years old. She arrived home from school one afternoon to find that her treasured border collie, Pasja, was gone. Her mother announced, "I don't like dogs," and that was that. Pasja was no more.

The loss was stark and crushing. And it was profoundly unnerving. If Pasja could disappear like that, what else could? What other people or things from her life could be whisked away without notice? What other givens could unhinge without warning?

Young Corine became cautious and guarded. Coming home from school was always fraught with tension because Corine never knew what to expect. Her mother's moods would shift precipitously: She could be bed-bound one day, frenetic the next. Some days she was hardly responsive, other days she was physically violent. On occasion she would be waiting for Corine with fragrant homemade tomato soup. At that age, Corine didn't know anything about depression or suicidality, but she instinctively knew to be wary. She didn't

understand why this was all happening, but she knew she was somehow the cause.

And she never, ever brought friends home to play.

When she was sixteen, her father was diagnosed with a brain
tumor. Melanoma had metastasized to his brain and he was suddenly
gravely ill and in need of intensive medical care. Corine's mother
was incapable of handling the medical issues, so Corine was left to
navigate this largely on her own. She recalls that the doctors spoke
mostly in euphemisms, which infuriated her. She couldn't stand the
condescending attitude that adults seemed to adopt whenever they
dealt with younger people. "Your father is very ill," the doctor had
said to her, "and we will have to remove some things from his body."

"Things? What things?" she snapped. "You mean the tumor in his
head?" The doctor was taken aback by the directness of this teenager.
He backpedaled, obfuscating even more. Corine was baffled and
insulted by the doctor's opaqueness. Even after the brain mass was
removed, the doctor still talked about the "peanut" that was taken
out of her father's head. When her father was discharged home, Corine discovered he could hardly take care of himself and often didn't
recognize who she was. Several times he wandered off during the
night. For weeks, sixteen-year-old Corine floundered in this unten-
able situation, struggling to manage a father who was now like an
advanced Alzheimer's patient and a mother who was enveloped by
her own demons. In desperation she marched back to the hospital
and told the doctors she was unable to take care of her father. He was
readmitted to the hospital and died there within the month, not even
a year from the initial melanoma diagnosis.

Now it was just Corine and her mother—the wary and the unstable. The years that followed were difficult, angry years. There were
days Corine needed to run away from the house to be safe. She finally left the turmoil of her home at age twenty-one, ready to be
done and gone. As she walked out the door, her mother bade her
good-bye with "You are no longer my child."

Corine moved, however, into more turmoil. She married a man
with extensive medical issues, and for the six years of their marriage,
he was in and out of hospitals. Corine had a front-row seat, however

unpleasant, in the theater of the health-care system. Many things upset her, but one of the most profound observations was that although the doctors were the experts, she—the spouse—often knew much more about the patient than they did. But as the spouse, she wasn't considered an expert. She was just "the family" of the patient.

When Corine was twenty-nine her mother was diagnosed with stomach cancer. It had been more than a decade since her father's metastatic melanoma, and Corine was now much more savvy about medicine than she'd been at sixteen. The cancer wasn't curable but the doctor informed Corine that her mother would undergo chemotherapy that would extend her life. Corine said, "Did you ask my mother if she actually wants the treatment?"

"Well, of course she should get treated," the doctor responded sharply. "She's only sixty-two years old and would respond well to the treatment. This would give her more time."

What, Corine wondered, would "responding well" actually mean? She knew her mother's life was miserable; her depression was intractable, and she was in and out of psych wards. All those suicide attempts were a clear message: she did not want to live this life. Why would she want more time? "Ask her," Corine said wearily to the doctor. "Just *ask* her."

So the doctor did, and was shocked when the patient gave a flat-out no. He was flabbergasted that an otherwise healthy sixty-two-year-old woman might decline treatment that would extend her life. Corine didn't wish for her mother's death, but she remembers saying to her grandmother, "This war will finally come to an end." Six weeks later, her mother died quietly, finally at peace with herself and the world.

Corine studied communications and had become interested in the field of mediation, how people could settle conflicts without the grueling antagonism that court cases usually entailed. It was obvious, of course, that the trick to being a good mediator was listening. But more important, it was recognizing each person's reality. As a child, her survival depended on intuiting her mother's perspective. Even if her mother's perspective was delusional, that perspective was the reality that her mother was operating from. In the cold calculus of survival, her mother's reality was the only one that counted, even if it was out of sync with actual reality. And so young Corine had honed these unusual battle skills, each day piecing together her mother's idiosyncratic reality, decoding and adapting to the erratic rules of engagement. It required paying careful attention to the most minute and subtle details.

When the adult Corine thought about the process of mediation, she realized that the way to successfully defuse conflicts was to similarly elucidate each party's reality. And the best way to accomplish this was to keep your own mouth shut and to listen—deeply, thoroughly, and attentively. She ended up being hired as the head of communications for a regional broadcasting station. Corine was tasked with coming up with a plan to improve their ratings, so she asked the director, "Who is your audience?" To her surprise, he really didn't know.

She could have mailed out a typical corporate survey but she figured she'd end up with generic data about age, income, marital status. She decided instead to visit the listeners in their homes. She quickly discovered that people were delighted to talk, both about the music they enjoyed and their lives in general.

These conversations lasted an hour or more. Each person had a unique and interesting story, and Corine was endlessly intrigued. There were days when she ended up spending an entire afternoon with a family, mainly listening, as people unspooled their lives, opening up their worlds to her. Around this time, she'd begun dabbling with social media. Her fascination with these listening experiences was the main subject of her nascent online writing ventures.

At the farthest-east border of Gelderland province sits Radboud University Medical Center. It's so close to the national border that an errant left turn will put you in Germany. The name of the province, in fact, comes from the German city of Geldern—a stone's throw away—which had functioned as the regional seat of this section of the Roman Empire. The city of Nijmegen, where Radboud hospital is located, dates from the Roman era (in 2005 it celebrated its two thousandth birthday). Radboud is one of the largest hospitals in the Netherlands, but at the time that Corine Jansen was working for the provincial radio station, the hospital was in crisis. Just a few years earlier its cardiothoracic surgery unit had been summarily shut down after a spate of deaths highlighted mortality rates that were three times the national average. A new CEO promptly sacked all of the department heads. The surgery unit was painstakingly restructured and eventually reopened but there was a general feeling that the hospital had lost its way.

Lucien Engelen had been hired to figure out the problems and help re-create the hospital in a way that would work more successfully. In essence, he was being asked to reshape the entire hospital. Thus was created the new REshape Innovation Center, and he was placed in charge. Lucien stumbled across Corine's posts on Twitter about her experiences listening in the homes of the broadcast customers. He wrote to her and offered her a job on the spot. "What's the job called?" Corine asked.

"I don't know," Lucien answered. He paused. "How about 'Chief Listening Officer?'" Chief Listening Officer was a job title pioneered by Kodak and Dell. The word "listening," though, was somewhat metaphorical. The role of Chief Listening Officer in these institutions was to pay attention to what the public was posting online about their companies. Chief "Paying Attention" Officer probably would have been a more accurate title, but it obviously lacked the necessary corporate snap. Whatever the title, these folks were incredibly successful helping the companies understand what their customers needed, and Lucien wanted to replicate that. Corine, however, was interested in *actual* listening. She wanted to listen to real people in their real-life worlds.

Lucien was intrigued by her approach. He recognized that if his hospital really wanted to solve its problems, it needed to hear the observations and opinions of *all* of the people involved in making a hospital function: doctors, nurses, patients, families, orderlies, housekeepers, administrators, technicians, therapists.

Within twenty-four hours Corine quit her job in broadcasting and signed on. The crispness of her career change, though, did not necessarily mask her mixed feelings about the health-care system. Having wrestled with the system during her father's struggle with and death from melanoma, her mother's borderline personality disorder and gastric cancer, her former husband's illness, and her own health issues, she knew all too well that navigating hospitals was a lot more fraught than figuring out which radio station on the dial you wanted to listen to.

One of the first assignments that fell into Corine's lap as Chief Listening Officer came from the oncology department. One segment of that department's patient population was especially vocal with its complaints: the young adult group. Of the two thousand cancer patients ages eighteen to thirty-five in the Netherlands, a full quarter of them were being treated at Radboud University Medical Center. They filed complaints about the food, the service, the decor, the wait times. They seemed reasonably satisfied with the medical care itself, but with everything else, the hospital just couldn't seem to get it right.

Corine used the same approach as she had with the radio station listeners. She didn't send out surveys or even invite the patients to her office to talk. Rather, she contacted them and offered to visit wherever they were—in their homes, at work, in the chemotherapy suite, at their doctor appointments, with their families, with their friends. They would talk for an hour or two, sometimes three. Occasionally Corine spent a whole afternoon with them, observing how they navigated their lives both inside and outside the hospital, listening to their observations about what was going well and what wasn't.

She didn't bring a prepared battery of questions. The only thing she asked, when the moment felt right, was whether the patients would feel comfortable telling her their story. If they did, she asked them to describe it from day one, from the very first moment they noticed a twinge in some nether region of their body or were informed that something was amiss in a blood test, up until the present. Like the radio station listeners, the patients were eager to talk. Walking down the antiseptic linoleum of a hospital corridor, or sunk into the comfortable concavities of a living room couch, or over a crisp Tripel Karmeliet beer with *ossenworst* sausage in a café, Corine listened.

She heard about the first symptoms, the first visit to a GP, and the rounds of labs and tests. There was the first nervous visit to an oncologist, the first tense trip to the hospital, the first nerve-wracking surgery, the first apprehensive round of chemotherapy or radiation. Corine also heard the stories told by the patients' families, friends, and co-workers, learning how cancer drove its spiny tentacles into an ever-widening network.

Corine had expected to hear mostly about cancer, and there was certainly a lot about that: patients described how their lives had abruptly pitched from ordinary to chaotic. They described a pressure cooker of fear and anxiety. But in many cases the cancer was the easy part because the medical teams offered plenty of information about that. But there wasn't anyone anywhere offering advice on whether it was okay to have sex. Nobody was helping them with how best to tell colleagues at work, or how to reconfigure university exams to accommodate chemotherapy. There were millions of details involved in knitting cancer and its endless unwanted baggage into everyday life, but patients and families were largely left to muddle through on their own.

After weeks of interviews, Corine closed her office door and wrote up the stories of two dozen of these young patients. When she was done, she sent them to the chief of oncology and the CEO of the hospital. Within twenty minutes she received a reply. "How much money do you need?" the CEO asked her. "Please don't stop listening to our patients."

I first met Corine over coffee on a mild June afternoon when she was visiting New York City. I could see instantly why people would open up unreservedly to tell their stories to her. There is something so obviously receptive about her, with her soft, open face, ever-welcoming smile, sunny disposition, and eyes that crinkle thoughtfully as she listens. Her wispy blond hair shifts to the side as she cocks her head ever so slightly when you are talking. She makes you feel like she genuinely wants to hear what you have to say, which isn't hard because she genuinely does. In our society today, we're so used to an underlying agenda being strapped to nearly every interaction that Corine's absolute lack of artifice can be disarming. Here is someone who feels that right now your story is the most important thing in the world and is prepared to sit with you for as long as it takes to tell it. Eyes aren't flitting to the clock or to a phone or to other people in the room. Her gaze and her entire posture are focused entirely on you.

We spoke for more than an hour that day, and then several more times by phone. Each time I felt as though we could talk endlessly. Every question she asked me made it clear that she'd been listening meticulously to what I'd been saying. That stimulated me to think very hard about my answers, and to come up with thoughtful questions for her. Even when she asked me to decelerate my barreling New York speaking pace—which she had to do frequently, but oh so politely—it felt like a compliment. I got the sense she was determined not to miss anything.

Being listened to so attentively is a remarkably energizing experience. It makes you eager to continue engaging. It also makes you feel refreshingly valued and respected: what you are saying is important. None of this is rocket science, but in an age of fragmented focus, limited attention spans, absurd levels of multitasking, and the annoying interference of technology, being intensely listened to for an extended period of time is a singular experience, one that leaves you in a better place than when you started. "When people talk, listen completely," wrote Ernest Hemingway, giving advice to a young writer. Given all that Hemingway was able to mine from the human experience, it's advice that would apply equally to the medical field.

Corine spent six years as the Chief Listening Officer at Radboud hospital. After the oncology project, she was asked to help with the issue of medical error. Patients who'd just experienced errors were, understandably, in a jumble of emotions. They were upset, angry, frightened, confused. They were worried about their health, unsure if they should call a lawyer, often wondering if they could ever trust their doctors or the hospital again. Equally potent emotions were roiling within the staff members who had been involved with the error: shame, guilt, embarrassment, confusion.

Corine was called in to listen to each person involved—the patients, family members, doctors, nurses, administrators. Listening was her only job; she wasn't asked to help the parties negotiate, or to provide advice, or even to be a therapist. Just to listen. No miracles ensued from the listening, but as everyone individually unloaded their stories, the air would usually begin to clear. The tension would start to dissipate and the parties could begin to move forward. Whether moving forward meant a settlement, or a plan for how to prevent the error in the future, or just a straightforward apology, or a full-blown lawsuit—typically these actions came about with less friction because each party had been fully heard.

As word spread in the hospital that this dynamic Chief Listening Officer was available, doctors began to request her when a difficult situation arose with a patient. Patients began requesting her when they were unsure how to proceed with their medical decision-making. Families began requesting her when there was confusion or tension in the air. Each time she used the same approach—attentive listening, the occasional question for clarification, and full-throttle attention. "Often I didn't even speak at all," Corine told me. The sessions would last until the person had finished saying everything they needed to say, usually for an hour, sometimes two. She didn't dispense advice or opinions. Occasionally a patient would ask her to convey a particular bit of the story to the doctor, but otherwise she just listened.

For six years Corine commuted three hours a day back and forth to Radboud Hospital. It was an exciting job, but the travel was beginning to exhaust her and she had her own health issues to contend with. Her doctors finally recommended that she cut back on her travel, so Corine reluctantly resigned from her position.

But Radboud Hospital had indeed reshaped itself over the years that Corine was there. Patients are now involved in advisory groups for every part of the health-care process, and many are active in co-creating programs with the hospital staff. Any new hospital initiative requires approval by the patient advisory board. Listening has become ingrained in Radboud's culture, and the hospital even hosted the first European Listening and Healthcare Conference. Medical care has improved and the hospital consistently ranks at the top of the ratings for health-care quality in Europe.

Corine is now an independent consultant, helping hospitals, medical schools, nursing homes, and clinics incorporate active listening into their daily operations. She also helps patients sort out their own stories. She is aware that a typical doctor's visit doesn't allow the luxury of a full hour for listening, so she helps patients shape their story into a concise three-minute narrative that they can bring to the appointment. She helps them prioritize what they need the doctor to know and what can wait for a follow-up visit.

Corine is bent on humanizing health care, and is convinced that listening is an enormously powerful tool. She certainly doesn't shy away from technology—she maintains an active social media presence—but observes that technology often ends up detracting from listening. "These technologies often become their own goal," she notes, "rather than a means to advance health care." She sees "live care" as embodying the quality of being human, and listening as a key means of fortifying that sense of humanness—something that often seems under attack in twenty-first-century medicine.

Recently, the Dutch government approved an insurance code for listening—that is, doctors can include listening as a legitimate part of the medical visit, on par with procedures and tests. You might think that listening already is a sine qua non of a doctor's visit, but because it wasn't possible to bill for it, procedures and tests naturally took precedence. Saying that a doctor's visit that consists entirely of talking and listening is as worthy of reimbursement as an endoscopy or MRI is a big step. This has been immensely validating for Corine, as she sees it is a cornerstone of high-quality health care. So far it's only for listening to patients' end-of-life concerns. "But it's a start," Corine says, with characteristic optimism. Soon maybe insurance companies will recognize that listening to the patient *before* the end of life is equally important, and can result in tangible medical benefits.

CHAPTER 8

Listen to Me

"I would be careful," a fellow physician warned Juliet Mavromatis when she told him about her plans to attend the birthday party of her patient Morgan Amanda Fritzlen. While not considered unethical, friendships between doctors and patients are viewed as a gray area, with the potential for clouding judgment from either perspective. Many physicians are extremely leery about any connection at all with patients outside the office. But Juliet was acutely aware that the working relationship she had with Morgan Amanda wasn't smooth. Though they got along in a personable fashion, there were still ongoing clashes between them about high-risk treatments that Morgan Amanda was insisting on. A doctor-patient relationship couldn't survive on amiable pleasantries alone. Plus, Juliet was genuinely interested in Morgan Amanda as a person.

The daughter of (and granddaughter of and eventually sister of) cultural anthropologists, Juliet spent childhood summers in a remote Brazilian fishing village. Her father toted her and her brother along as he did fieldwork, spending hours in deep conversation with local residents to learn about their lives and earn their trust. At age fifteen Juliet and her family moved from their quiet Midwestern college town to the flamboyance of Rio de Janeiro for a year.

Growing up in this unusual anthropological cauldron engendered in Juliet a genuine curiosity and respect for the tapestries of her patients' lives. "I decided that if Morgan Amanda was to trust me," Juliet told me, "I had to take a different approach. I had been fighting with her over the direction of her medical care but didn't want to continue that way; I would have to connect on another level."

Morgan Amanda was actually thinking the same thing. She liked Juliet as a person, but she was frustrated by Juliet's reservations about every aspect of the treatment. She was also painfully aware that she was entirely dependent upon Juliet—no other doctor had been willing to take her case and no other doctor would write the orders for the cyclophosphamide treatment so that she could remain in the Emory health-care system. But she needed more than a doctor who was just agreeable; she needed a passionate advocate. When Morgan Amanda invited Juliet to the party celebrating her twenty-second birthday, she was seeking to strengthen their relationship and Juliet's commitment.

The party took place on a blazingly hot and humid July afternoon, just shy of the one-year mark of their doctor-patient relationship. The magnolia trees had long since shed their incandescent pink and white flowers, and were now just part of the lush Georgia greenery that enlivened the windows of the thankfully air-conditioned party room. The mood of the well-wishers matched the overabundance of food: curries, biryanis, sushi, plus plenty of "plain food" for guests with less-adventurous palates. Juliet felt like an honored guest as Morgan Amanda introduced her around to her family, friends, and teachers.

The pièce de résistance was the birthday cake that Morgan Amanda's mother had topped with a painted glass peacock ornament, complete with brilliant willowy feathers. It was so stunning that Morgan Amanda saved it and hung it on her Christmas tree every year thereafter. Morgan Amanda looked radiant in her cream-colored dress with its hexagonal accents of navy blue and deep yellow. She chatted with the guests, making sure everyone had enough to eat and someone to talk to, occasionally swiping off the vanilla frosting from her slice of cake. (Morgan Amanda was generally health conscious in her eating habits, but frosting was her one weak spot. She'd buy it by the can—the cheapest and junkiest she could find—and polish it off with a spoon.)

Juliet gave a gift of her favorite book, *The Fountainhead*. ("I love it for the characters, not the politics!" Juliet hastened to tell me.) For Morgan Amanda it was a moment of uncommon linkage, because *The Fountainhead* was also her father's favorite book.

After the party, the doctor-patient relationship took on a distinctly different quality. Morgan Amanda shared some of her personal writings with Juliet, as well as her dream of going to medical school. "We bonded on a number of things," Juliet recalled. "Writing, medicine, books . . . shoes. I think we might have been friends if we'd met in another setting."

While their relationship improved, Morgan Amanda's health, unfortunately, did not. The cyclophosphamide, which helped initially, did not turn out to be a panacea. The illness flared up with a vengeance. As the trees unfurled their palettes of mahogany and gold, Morgan Amanda became plagued with worsening weakness, fatigue, fevers, sweating, joint pains, and swollen legs. She landed in the ER several times, as doctors tried to tease out whether she was experiencing blood clots, infections, or her "regular" arthritis. She became weaker and sicker. By Thanksgiving she was barely able to walk with crutches. Her weight dropped to ninety-eight pounds, her body almost a billowing sheet on her six-foot frame.

"I spiraled into a crater of illness," Morgan Amanda said. "I was sicker than I'd ever been. I was afraid to make the declaration that cyclophosphamide wasn't working because there was nothing to take after cyclophosphamide." Cyclophosphamide was the end of the line, and everyone knew it. Morgan Amanda was beginning to feel hopeless. Medically, she was desperate.

Experimental treatments were considered. Her hematologist suggested plasmapheresis—a complete filtering of the blood to remove antibodies. Her psychiatrist prescribed antidepressants but these served to exacerbate her shakiness and sweats. The worsening shakes and sweats were thought to be symptomatic of panic attacks, so tranquilizers were prescribed. Opiates were added for the unremitting pain. The number of medications and their possible interactions and side effects was staggering.

Meanwhile Morgan Amanda was combing the Internet for new treatments. She stumbled upon a few experimental trials in which bone marrow transplants were being tested for autoimmune diseases and began to pursue the possibility of this treatment.

The next medical appointment, in early December, was what both doctor and patient would refer to as the "critical point" in their relationship. Morgan Amanda was still taking cyclophosphamide, afraid to stop it, even though by this point it clearly wasn't working. She'd been talking with her rheumatologist about a bone marrow transplant, but meanwhile the cyclophosphamide orders needed to be renewed every month. For that, she needed Juliet.

The visit was late in the day, a last-minute add-on appointment. Juliet had been pondering Morgan Amanda's case, concerned about her worsening condition and the escalating side effects of the medications. Juliet sought the advice of several experienced clinicians at Emory. Each expressed utter disbelief at Juliet's prescribing such a high-risk medical regimen that ran counter to her own clinical judgment. Juliet found herself increasingly worried, not just about the medicolegal ramifications, but that she could be directly harming her patient.

The visit began with the usual opening pleasantries. In most of their visits Morgan Amanda was the one who took the lead in the conversation, usually with a bullet list of items to discuss. But this visit was different, with Juliet taking a firm lead.

"I want to talk to you about the cyclophosphamide," Juliet said, sitting in her chair while Morgan Amanda perched on the exam table. "You've been e-mailing me about renewing the orders but it is clear that the medication is not working. I spoke to your rheumatologist over the weekend and told him how uncomfortable this makes me. I worry that I am harming you by prescribing this."

Morgan Amanda was already in a tense state. She was sicker than she'd ever been, worried she was running out of treatment options. She felt strung out on all the psychiatric medications that had been piled onto her regimen. She'd been waiting nervously in the waiting room for more than an hour before she'd been called in to the exam room. Her hackles were already raised. When Juliet made this statement, Morgan Amanda did not hear concern; she heard that her doctors were talking about her behind her back.

Juliet continued calmly but definitively. "I've felt conflicted about writing these orders all along; I've never heard of any other primary-care doctor prescribing such a toxic drug as cyclophosphamide. And it isn't even clear to me that rheumatoid arthritis is what is causing all your symptoms. I'm not convinced that this is your true diagnosis."

Intellectually, Morgan Amanda knew that Juliet was pointing out what they all knew—that her symptoms did not fit the classic RA picture, that the drugs were not working—but psychologically she heard "You're not really sick." Juliet's doubting of the RA diagnosis was, in effect, undermining the very framework that enabled Morgan Amanda to receive care. For someone who had been doubted all along, who'd had to fight to get care, who'd had to face the fact that most doctors did not want to touch her case, this sounded like "There's nothing wrong with you."

Morgan Amanda abruptly catapulted herself off the exam table, her frustrations of the past year boiling over and her words erupting with uncharacteristic vitriol and barely suppressed tears. "Why now? Why do you suddenly have a decisive opinion now?" The sobs intensified. "*I've* been doing your job most of the time—all the research, coordination, negotiations. I have to figure everything out for my care and stay on your case to get things done. Why *now* do you want to step in and take decisive action? Why do you suddenly care to do something now?"

Juliet was taken aback by the firestorm and endeavored to keep things from escalating. "I do care," she said quietly, while Morgan Amanda hovered above her, unsteady on her feet. "I care very much. That is why I'm telling you that the cyclophosphamide treatment seems to be doing more harm than good. In fact, I've had dreams—*nightmares*—that you died from the medications I'm prescribing."

For Morgan Amanda these admissions did not come across as signs of caring; they felt paternalistic. *If you really cared*, she thought, *you would understand that I need someone to push the boundaries. If you really cared, you would be aggressively hunting down other treatments, not jumping ship when one drug isn't working.* Years later she was able to accept that Juliet really did care and was in a tough spot, but at the time she heard her doctor backing out. *I'm gutsier than this woman,* she thought. *I'm willing to fight for my life.* So she brought up the issue of the bone marrow transplant.

Juliet had heard about this from the rheumatologist, but this was the first time Morgan Amanda had brought it up with her. Chemotherapy agents such as rituximab and cyclophosphamide were one thing, but a bone marrow transplant was in a different stratosphere. Used typically with lymphomas, leukemias, and other cancers, the procedure involves obliterating a patient's own bone marrow with high-dose chemotherapy and radiation, destroying all native red cells, white cells, and platelets. Then, stem cells from a donor are transplanted.

Destroying the bone marrow, by definition, decimates the body's immune system, leaving a person vulnerable to deadly infections, not to mention blood clots, intestinal breakdown, and liver failure. Yes, the "rebooting" of the immune system offered the theoretical possibility of curing Morgan Amanda's autoimmune illness, not to mention her life-threatening allergic reactions, but the risks were immense. Death was a distinct possibility.

Even though Juliet knew this might be coming, she was nevertheless almost too dumbfounded to speak when the topic came up. "Do you have any idea of what a bone marrow transplant entails? It could *kill* you."

"I know what a bone marrow transplant entails," Morgan Amanda snapped, leaning unsteadily on a crutch. She could feel her body shaking with anger as she started jamming papers and books into her purse. She avoided making eye contact with Juliet because she knew that it would open the floodgates. She was desperate not to break down completely in front of her doctor.

Juliet pressed on, pulling out her armamentarium of facts. "And a doctor can't just 'write an order' for a bone marrow transplant. It's an enormous process. Plus, I've never even *heard* of bone marrow transplants being used for RA." It was already growing dark outside and this visit was wearing Juliet down—both physically and emotionally. How much longer could it go on like this? But she had to say what she was really feeling. "The bigger point," she said, "is that we don't really know what disease you have. To consider such a serious treatment with an unclear diagnosis is not just dangerous, it's *reckless*."

To Morgan Amanda, this was the last straw. All of her other treatment options had failed and her body was slowly giving way. Juliet's jettisoning of the bone marrow transplant idea was tantamount to abandonment. "That's it! I'm done," she burst out. "I'm done and I'm leaving. I'm finished with this." She stormed out of Juliet's office, or at least stormed as much as she could—heaving her skeletal body onto the crutches, slinging her bulging purse that was heavy enough to ballast a battleship, and hobbling out the door, by now crying too hard to even see where she was going.

"It truly felt like my doctor was abandoning me," Morgan Amanda said later, "both medically and personally." There was no way she could continue to work with Juliet. She was ready to fire her doctor.

As it happened, Juliet was thinking the exact same thing about Morgan Amanda. After that draining visit Juliet sat down and wrote a letter to her patient, formally resigning as her physician. Their interactions were taking such an emotional toll that she felt she could no longer effectively be Morgan Amanda's doctor.

But the letter was never sent.

What is so striking about the conversation between Morgan Amanda and Juliet is the mismatch between what each person said and what the other person heard. Over the course of a year, I spoke extensively with Juliet and with Morgan Amanda about their time together. Both women approached their recollections thoughtfully and intelligently, willing to self-reflect and take responsibility for their own shortcomings. Both were remarkably generous in spirit—to themselves and to the other person. Both expressed genuine respect and obvious fondness for the other.

But even with that, it sometimes felt as though they were telling two different stories. Even accounting for vagaries of memory and differing points of view, it was clear they'd drawn different conclusions from the same set of events.

What patients say and what doctors hear can be two very dissimilar things. The reverse is also quite true: what doctors say and what patients hear can be radically different. When Juliet confronted her patient about the side effects of cyclophosphamide and the excessiveness of considering a bone marrow transplant, Morgan Amanda didn't hear it as a medical discussion of risks and benefits. She heard a doctor denying that she was sick, another doctor getting ready to walk away from her care. With hindsight, as well as a particular strength of character, Morgan Amanda could recognize that Juliet was genuinely trying to do the right thing as a physician, that Juliet really *was* thinking about her patient's health and trying to prioritize it. But at the time, in that particular context, with the physical and emotional stakes so high, she could not hear that.

Juliet was also able to eventually recognize what she was not able to hear in the moment. "From her standpoint," Juliet later wrote to me in a letter, "her quality of life was very poor, and she was willing to take huge risks in an attempt to improve it. Perhaps I never could fully understand this perspective."

Listening is one of the most intricate skills we possess, yet also one that seems so obvious that we hardly ever think about it. It's like walking—no one ever laid out the instruction manual for you, but you somehow know how to do it. Even though we may hear what people say without exerting any effort, how we extract information from what's being spoken (and how we convey that understanding) is another ballgame altogether.

If you are sitting in a lecture hall, for example, and a professor is droning on about fifteenth-century religious tractates, or pyruvate kinase activity in the mitochondria, or moral symbolism in *Silas Marner*, your brain could very well be in a passive mode. Sounds and words float in—a few stick, most drift distractedly away. Or someone is speaking right at you but your mind is focused on your snarling stomach and its misguided choice of deep-fried burrito, or your tenuously napping baby in the next room, or that locust of a phone buzzing in your back pocket. You are preoccupied and only vaguely catching what might be the most scintillating conversation since Lincoln debated Douglas.

By contrast, it's quite different when you determinedly strive to listen to what is being said—instructions on cashing in your winning lottery ticket, for example, or a declaration of love from someone you could possibly love back, or the moment you recognize that pyruvate kinase catalyzes the production of ATP, which is the gasoline that powers the cell and so by definition powers the entire body, and that is perhaps the coolest thing you ever possibly could imagine and to hell with a career in medicine and your student loans and your parents' expectations, you're going to become a biochemist and squeak by from grant to grant and live in a ratty lab coat as long as it gets you into the lab and into those miraculous cells.

In these cases, you invest your energy into hearing every word and extracting meaning from those words, even meaning that resides between the lines. Such active listening requires intense focus—on the person speaking, on the words being spoken, and on the nonverbal cues that clarify meaning. But these concepts of passive and active listening embody only part of the multidimensionality of listening. There is a whole academic field that studies listening as a relational activity, something that creates a relationship between two people.

"Extracting information," says Graham Bodie, a listening researcher from Louisiana State University, "is too simplistic a definition of listening. It presumes that talking is a linear process, that words are a mere conduit with meaning packed inside, that the listener just needs to unpack them at the other end, like opening a letter." This concrete portrayal of communication may have come about because of a quirk of history in which communications research arose from the field of public speaking rather than from academia. As Bodie described it, underappreciated English teachers in the early 1900s formed the first organization dedicated to teaching proper public speaking. At the time, public speaking was considered the epitome of communication, and so the premise of early communication theory was that the speaker at the podium would gather the pertinent facts into a tidy bundle and dispatch it off to the listener in the audience like a basket on a zip line.

"Unfortunately," Bodie says, "this places a large burden on the speaker." To improve communication, the speaker needs to be clearer, or more expressive, or employ superior words, or simply holler louder. The listener, by contrast, has only to sit back and wait for the speaker to compose the most efficacious basket of facts and sail it forward.

Indeed, this is how doctor-patient communication is often viewed. The burden is on the patient to tell the clearest, most informative story so the doctor can make the appropriate diagnosis. In a teaching hospital, after an intern takes a medical history from a patient, the intern then presents that history to the rest of the medical team on rounds. The intern may preface this presentation—which typically is out of earshot of the patient—by noting that the patient is a "poor historian." This is not (usually) said in a derogatory way, but rather expressed as an objective fact to inform others on the team that the story is going to be a bit patchy because the patient didn't know many of the medical details.

Aside from the faintly ridiculous nature of the terminology—I'll often wonder aloud to the intern whether perhaps that patient might make a better sociologist or archeologist—there is the implicit reminder, once again, that the full responsibility for effective communication is on the speaker, in this case that shifty, unreliable patient. So if the medical history presented on rounds is a muddled mess, it's not because of the intern's lack of effective listening or preparation. It's because the patient wasn't clear enough, or organized enough, or smart enough, or thorough enough, or loud enough. But, Bodie says, "both people are equally responsible. They co-create the meaning."

Janet Bavelas, a Canadian researcher at the University of Victoria, conducted a set of ingenious experiments to illustrate this.[1] She and her colleagues studied student volunteers who were paired up as speakers and listeners. The speakers had to tell detailed, dramatic stories about near misses or close calls in their own lives. The listeners had to, well, listen. Some of the listeners, however, were told that while the speaker was telling the story, they were to count in their head the number of official holidays (no-school days) from now until Christmas. The experiment was conducted in February so there were a fair number of holidays to account for. In a second version of the experiment, some listeners were instructed to press a button every time the speaker used a word starting with the letter "t."

Unsurprisingly, the holiday counters weren't very good listeners. They exhibited many fewer of the generic indicators of paying attention: saying "mm-hmm" or "yeah," or nodding. And they showed hardly any specific responses—gestures or expressions that reflected the actual content of the story.

We are very familiar with the holiday counters, people with that semi-glazed look while listening. We know they are thinking about their to-do list, or last night's to-the-buzzer basketball game, or whether the minestrone soup will run out by the time they get to the cafeteria, rather than focusing on what we are saying.

What I found interesting about this study was the use of the second type of distracted listener, the t-word counters. Unlike the holiday counters, these listeners had to focus extremely attentively on the speakers in order to catch those t-words. These listeners were able to provide the typical generic responses, nodding at the right time, saying "mm-hmm" at the right time. But it turns out they were equally lousy at giving any specific responses. That is, although they were listening attentively, they weren't actually *hearing* the story being told.

But the most surprising effect of the two types of distraction was not on the listener, but on the speaker. When the listeners were not attentive, the speakers faltered at the climaxes of their stories. Their stories became choppier, more run-on, with extra filler words and awkward pauses. Sometimes the speaker ended up circling around and giving the ending again, or explaining and justifying the climax. (Remember, these were personal close-call stories that by definition were dramatic for the storyteller.)

I expected that the holiday counters would have caused more discombobulation in the speakers than the t-word counters, as they were off on a completely extraneous tangent, but in fact the experiment showed the exact opposite. It was the t-word counters who threw off the speakers the most. It may have been that the speakers could see that the holiday counters were obviously disengaged and so tuned them out as lost causes. But the t-word counters were tricky—they *seemed* engaged but actually weren't. They appeared to be focusing hard on the listener but weren't actually hearing the story, so their responses were mismatched both in timing and in appropriateness. This can be very disconcerting to the speaker, who can't figure out if the story is connecting. The speaker ends up stumbling in the telling, saddled with a dramatic personal story that now seems sort of ridiculous, floundering about to end in a respectable manner.

This study demonstrates the crucial role the listener plays in the quality of the speaker's story. The listener is coaxing the story to life. The better listener—the one who is paying attention to the story and letting the speaker know about that attention—helps the speaker deliver a smooth, logical, and compelling story. Bavelas titled her paper about these experiments "Listeners as Co-Narrators." Gone is the standard idea of the listener merely slitting open the verbal bundle into which the speaker has dutifully packed his or her story. The listener is in fact a key element of the speaker's ability to tell an effective story. With appropriate responses that are specific to the content of the story, the listener helps draw out the story, helps illustrate the story, and even helps shape that story into its best possible form.

If it seems odd to have the listener "shaping" the speaker's story—this could be either cooperative or manipulative, depending on your point of view—think of what it's like to speak to someone who is unable to respond. Perhaps you've visited an elderly relative with severe dementia in a nursing home or a comatose patient in a hospital. We're always instructed to talk normally because you never know how much the other person can hear or process, and we always want to err on the side of making contact. However, it is profoundly uncomfortable to speak without getting any response or indication of understanding. We may start out recounting a recent happening in our lives, or giving an update on all of the family members, but after a while we falter. We feel silly talking into thin air. Our stories seem pointless and very quickly a creeping embarrassment overtakes us. Even though we want to talk to our loved ones in the hope that they are hearing something or maybe just appreciating a familiar voice, most of us dwindle off. It's just too awkward.

"It's a cooperative process," Bavelas told me. "The speaker and listener roles alternate during the conversation. Each needs feedback from the other to know whether information is getting through."

Doctors are taught to summarize or paraphrase what a patient says and offer it back to the patient to check for accuracy. "This is thought of as a neutral process," said Bavelas, "but it's not." In her studies of psychotherapists,[2] she observed that therapists make specific choices when they paraphrase what patients say. They can downplay certain details and emphasize others. They may reframe what the patient has said, add their own observations, even omit certain parts altogether. This certainly puts a good deal of power in the hands of the listener, in this case the therapist. Good therapists are mindful of this, and do so responsibly. Doctors, though, don't spend nearly as much time as therapists reflecting on their communication skills and are not as skilled in using this "shaping" to its best effect.

When I read the research of Graham Bodie and Janet Bavelas, it resonated immediately with the communication challenges between doctors and patients that I'd been grappling with. We doctors complain a lot about patients being "poor historians" but have never really considered that our listening styles may be significant contributors to that poor historianship. After speaking with these researchers I tried to pay closer attention to my own interactions with patients. How effectively was I listening? How much—and how beneficially—was I shaping the patient's story, if at all?

Not long after I spoke with Janet Balevas, I had a visit with Ross Leonard. This was our third medical visit together. Mr. Leonard is a man in his forties who I'd describe as a jack-of-all-trades. He'd worked at various times in construction, trucking, real estate, and commercial fishing. He hailed originally from Cleveland but sported a transcontinental employment history. Our first visit, some months prior, had not gone very well. He was annoyed from the get-go, impatiently telling me of the abdominal pain he'd had for the past many years. He reeled off the CT scans, endoscopies, and MRIs that he'd had—none of which had provided an answer. He ticked off on his fingers all the different medications he'd taken—none of which worked sufficiently. He brought in stacks of blood test results—none of which were abnormal. "So what's going on?" he demanded within five minutes of the start of our visit. "Tell me why I'm having all this pain!" His pale, freckly skin was already reddened and leathered by his years of outdoor work, but he managed to redden even more when he pressed me on this.

I obviously was not the master diagnostician—or soothsayer—he was evidently hoping for because I was not able to come up with a quick and neat explanation for his pain. No matter what I said, or what approach I offered, he just kept demanding an answer that I could not give.

For complicated patients like this the best advice is to push aside the stacks of old records and start from the very beginning, taking a thorough and methodical history. At our second visit I attempted this, despite my trepidation regarding the black hole of time we could easily fall into. My concerns were well founded, as every question I asked resulted in a torrent of responses that ranged from the graphic details of his second colonoscopy to the medication recommended to him by the coroner in Vegas (which worked fantastically, until it didn't). In retrospect, I could see that I was desperately trying to shape Mr. Leonard's story. With each eruption of facts, I paraphrased back to him what I was hearing. But I made deliberate choices to emphasize what seemed relevant, and downplay or even omit what seemed further afield. (Pursuing how he came to be getting medical advice from the coroner in Vegas seemed like a low-yield avenue of diagnostic inquiry.)

Mr. Leonard, though, was not inclined toward the cooperative side of co-narrating. The more demanding he became, the more briskly I found myself slicing away at his story, trying to pin him down to the most basic, concrete facts. There was no Kumbaya moment of co-creating meaning. There was no harmonious synergy of our perspectives, just an ever sharper battling over the facts. Suffice it to say that visit number two did not go down in the annals of medicine as a paragon of doctor-patient communication.

So here we were at visit three, each of us eyeing the other warily. Mr. Leonard arrived with a list of demands, including a very specific brand of eye drops, an MRI of his abdomen—"and make sure it's *with contrast*, not without"—a letter for his employer saying he was too sick to work, and a prescription for Viagra. Before stepping off from the riverbank into what promised to be yet another estuary of exasperation, I tried to meditate on what I'd been learning from these communications researchers. Was there a way that I could be a more productive listener? Could I adapt my responses to Mr. Leonard in a manner that would make his story more coherent and meaningful? Could I adjust my reactions to create a more trusting environment in which his narrative might flourish?

Janet Bavelas had talked to me about the importance of "grounding," the periodic acknowledgment to the speaker that he or she is being heard.[3] This could be a nod of the head or saying "mm-hmmm." This could be repeating back a phrase just after it was spoken, or making a comment that indicates you understood what was just said. So I tried that with Mr. Leonard. After every few statements I made sure to let him know that I'd heard him, that I'd gotten it and was still on the same page with him. I kept good eye contact; I encouraged whenever I could.

But it didn't seem to be working. Mr. Leonard barreled forward like the eighteen-wheelers he used to drive, annoyed that I wasn't producing an answer for his abdominal pain, clearly determined to march onward until his four demands were met. When it comes to grounding, I learned, an additional step is needed. After the speaker has spoken and the listener acknowledges that the speaker has been heard and understood, the speaker needs to somehow acknowledge that acknowledgment.[4] This may sound like an incessant Mobius strip, but in most conversations this happens so instinctively that it's never even noticed. But with Mr. Leonard, it was not occurring and the absence was clearly felt. Because it wasn't occurring, we weren't actually having a conversation. Once one key element dropped away, the whole enterprise came toppling down. No wonder both of us were cranky by the end of the visit.

I finally gave up and switched from conversation mode to negotiation mode. I laid out my terms. I told Mr. Leonard I would write the letter to his boss but would not excuse him from work; I'd describe his medical issues but would not render judgment about his fitness to work. I'd write the prescriptions for the fancy eye drops and for the Viagra, but neither was likely covered by his insurance, so I told him he should be prepared for jaw-dropping costs at the pharmacy.

The MRI, however, I would not order. He'd had one in the past year that didn't show any pathology and there was no medical indication to order another. In fact, I told him, I would not order *any* further tests until he kept a detailed symptom diary that we could examine at the next visit. To my surprise, Mr. Leonard acceded, though reluctantly. He grudgingly agreed to the terms and we parted on a slightly less fractious note.

There is much that goes into effective communication, I was learning, though Mr. Leonard reminded me that it doesn't always go by the book. I loved the idea that a doctor and patient could be co-narrators in the story. It's an ideal that I want to strive for, but I also have to accept that the reality of doctors, patients, and illness is a lot more unwieldy. And if all else fails, there's always the coroner in Vegas.

But let's turn back to Morgan Amanda Fritzlen and her doctor, Juliet Mavromatis, who were on the verge of firing each other. The patient was determined to seek a bone marrow transplant for her worsening symptoms, and the doctor was horrified by this dangerous and medically reckless idea.

Morgan Amanda feverishly researched hospitals around the country that might consider her for a bone marrow transplant. But meanwhile something had to be done about her worsening weakness, fevers, pain, and joint swellings. The rheumatoid arthritis, or whatever her actual disease was, had wasted her down to skeletal proportions.

Because this was most likely some sort of autoimmune disease, the hematologist began plasmapheresis—a wholesale filtering of the entire blood system to remove harmful antibodies. Plasmapheresis is a stopgap measure, since the body continues to make antibodies. However, it can sometimes help during an acute flare-up of an autoimmune illness. Before plasmapheresis can even begin, though, a catheter must be surgically inserted into the subclavian vein, a major vein that runs under the collarbone. This is typically a straightforward procedure but nothing was ever typical or straightforward for Morgan Amanda.

In her weakened and malnourished state, her immune system could not fight off infections arising from the catheter placement and the hospital environment. Like an army of Civil War proportions, with one row of soldiers cresting the hill after another, the pathogens kept coming. All told, five waves of infection ravaged her body during that hospitalization, including the dreaded MRSA (methicillin-resistant staph aureus) and VRE (vancomycin-resistant enterococcus).

The infections decimated what little reserve she possessed. A feeding tube was inserted into her stomach because she couldn't eat. But in her hyperinflammatory state, her body couldn't absorb the nutritional formula, and so she continued to waste away. During this time, the Emory bone marrow transplant team came by to evaluate her as she had requested. But one look at her was all they needed. "A bone marrow transplant would kill you" was their blunt assessment.

Morgan Amanda confided to her hematologist that she could no longer work with Juliet and was planning to fire her as her primary-care doctor. "Don't make rash decisions while you are this sick," the hematologist told her. "It's obvious that Dr. Mavromatis cares about you." Everyone around her echoed this, advising her to ride it out with Juliet. The unspoken warning was "How are you ever going to find another doctor?"

But Morgan Amanda didn't want to be dependent on someone she couldn't completely trust. She described it to me as like being in a boat with someone who was rowing in the opposite direction.

Because of the hospitalist system at Emory, Juliet was not directing the medical care during this hospital admission, though she remained in continuous consultation with the inpatient team. Juliet visited her patient in the hospital shortly before Christmas. It was the first time they'd seen each other since the explosive meeting in Juliet's office three weeks prior. Neither acknowledged what had transpired. The visit was cordial but restrained. It was strictly business on both ends: just reviewing the plasmapheresis treatment plan. There was no physical contact—no physical exam, not even a handshake.

"I was so tired," Morgan Amanda remembered. "I had no bite left."

Juliet herself was wary. She was casing the situation, as she put it later, to see if it was possible for them to rebuild trust and work together, or whether she'd have to deliver the letter of resignation that still sat in her desk drawer.

Morgan Amanda reiterated that she felt the bone marrow transplant was something she needed to consider. She knew that plasmapheresis was only a temporizing measure, a raft that might keep her afloat for a bit but could not pull her out of the churning waters that were engulfing her. Weary desperation was palpable in her voice, and Juliet heard this.

Juliet still had strong doubts about the transplant option, even about the diagnosis of rheumatoid arthritis, but she chose not to voice them at this moment. She had voiced them before, and repeating them wasn't going to help. But she felt she'd done the right thing in her office three weeks before by stating her clear opinion to Morgan Amanda. She felt she owed her patient an honest opinion, no matter how much it conflicted with her patient's desires.

However, the truth was that Juliet and the medical profession didn't have any other treatments to offer. So instead, she voiced her support for the herculean efforts Morgan Amanda was investing. These were not platitudes; Juliet was immensely impressed by her patient's determination, and Morgan Amanda heard this.

Juliet also knew that Morgan Amanda—by sheer tenacity and perseverance—would get herself evaluated by a transplant program, with or without Juliet as her doctor. Although it was certainly tempting to wash her hands of the case completely, Juliet knew this would not be good medicine. It wasn't good medicine to force her patient to find a new doctor—a process that could take months or in this case even a year—and then to have that new doctor start from scratch. It was better medicine to remain at her side as her primary-care doctor, to work to regain her trust. Beyond that, it simply felt right to Juliet as a person. She was not one to walk away from a difficult situation, so she decided to give it another shot. The letter would remain in her drawer.

Morgan Amanda had heard about the transplant program at another hospital in Atlanta. Juliet offered to look into it and she did. She made several phone calls and spoke personally with members of the transplant team. And so when she called her patient to say that unfortunately they—like Emory—did not do transplants for autoimmune disease, Morgan Amanda nevertheless felt Juliet had given the boat a genuine stroke in her direction.

CHAPTER 9

Just the Facts, Ma'am

As we've seen already, the doctor-patient interaction incorporates aspects both tangible and intangible. The intangible parts—empathy, compassion, good listening, nonverbal behavior, trust, respect—are critical, though notoriously difficult to quantify. Despite that intangibility, it's clear that an entire medical interaction can collapse when those factors are lacking. But what about the tangible parts, the basic medical facts that need to travel between doctor and patient? How well does this transpire? Luckily, facts here are much more straightforward to study and there is a robust field of research on this.

Doctor-patient communication can be imagined as a two-way highway of information. Each person is endeavoring to convey information to the other. One of the most information-laden points of contact between doctor and patient is upon discharge from the hospital. There are medications to talk about, as well as follow-up appointments. There may be a special diet to follow and certain restrictions on activity. There are often follow-up tests and labs, plus referrals to specialists and physical therapy. Then, of course, there is the most basic information that patients ought to know: their diagnosis and the name of their doctor. Amazingly, even these can be poorly communicated.

In one study, fewer than half of patients being discharged could name their main diagnosis.[1] In another study, 73 percent of patients knew that there was one primary doctor in charge of their care, but only 18 percent could name him or her.[2] This study, additionally, polled the doctors. Two-thirds were confident that their patients knew their names—quite a contrast with the 18 percent of patients who could actually cite that name. An even larger percentage of doctors (77 percent) were confident that their patients knew their diagnoses. But only 58 percent of patients in this study could name said diagnosis.

How could patients not know their diagnosis or the name of their doctor? Seems hard to believe. But if you've ever been hospitalized, you know what a byzantine and surreal environment a hospital is, especially a large teaching hospital. The phrase "medical team" hardly does justice to the armada of people in white coats who traipse in and out of your room. There's the intern, who might be in your room the most, doing various and sundry tasks for your care. There's the resident who supervises the intern, but you may see her less. There's the attending physician, who is the senior doctor on your case. He is the one at the top of the chart and may be making the most decisions for you, but you may see him only briefly. The white coat who actually spends the most time in your room could be the lowly medical student, who has virtually no say in your care but the most time to sit and talk. Then there are the consultants from other specialties, and each consult team can come stocked with student, intern, resident, fellow, and attending. There are nurses and physical therapists and dietary aides and respiratory technicians and nutritionists and case managers—all of whom might be wearing white coats.

Even if all of these white coated folks conscientiously offer their name and role to you, and respectfully wear their ID card at your eye level with a large-size font thoughtfully selected by the hospital, it's difficult for even the most organized human being to keep track of who's who. Especially if you are flat on your back in bed, feeling rotten, in pain, possibly terrified, and receiving assorted medications that can make you dizzy, nauseated, itchy, gassy, or worse. But that doesn't mean it's impossible to adequately communicate under these conditions—it just means that we medical staff have to be more cognizant of the challenges.

An interesting comparison can be made right on the hospital ward. In a survey of 250 hospitalized patients, only 32 percent could name even *one* of their treating doctors. But 60 percent could correctly name their nurse.[3] This is a phenomenon that is well known in hospital corridors, and there are many possible reasons for this. Nurses tend to spend much more time in the rooms with patients than doctors do. Nurses are also much more likely to touch the patients, while doctors often stand at a distance and talk.

There isn't much research devoted to this topic, but when I posed the question to Theresa Brown, an oncology nurse and prominent writer in the health-care field, she agreed that nurses spend much more time in patient rooms than doctors do, which gives patients more time to talk with nurses. "In nursing school," she said, "we learn that the first chat of the shift is never just a chat but an opportunity to see how the patient is feeling, what their pain level is, whether they're eating, etc. We are taught that talking with patients is a crucial part of assessing them clinically."

This is quite different from medical school, in which doctors-to-be are taught to "take a history." Though both might ultimately yield the same information, there's a very different feel, and patients pick up on that.

"In general," Brown observed, "we nurses present ourselves as people to be talked to, whereas doctors often come across as people who do the talking." That distinction, I must say, gave me pause and some pangs of discomfort. Some of this imbalance may arise from patients being respectful to doctors, even deferential, but some may come from patients feeling intimidated. Intimidating patients is surely not the stated goal of most doctors, and it's upsetting to recognize that it still happens, even when we think we've moved permanently away from old-school paternalistic medicine.

But I also know the desperate feeling of having so much information to convey (in such a preposterously slender allotment of time) that I end up hammering one item after another after another. For patients receiving this information it is like drinking from a gushing hose—a torrent of information cascades at them and at best they can manage a handful of swallows.[4] Whether patients are leaving the hospital, the emergency room, or a regular office visit, less than half the information lobbed at them is typically retained.[5]

It's not that doctors don't think about this or try to improve communication, but the tools we use aren't necessarily the most effective. In one study, researchers dispatched a group of actors portraying patients into doctors' offices along with tape recorders.[6] The actors had been trained to offer the identical clinical presentation and background information, in this case about having gastric reflux symptoms. The researchers listened to the tapes and examined how the doctors attempted to convey information. The most common strategy was repetition. Doctors repeated information once, twice, sometimes three times. While repetition can enhance remembering, it can also come across as haranguing, especially if there is an element of guilt or discomfort involved (for example, reminding an overweight patient to avoid soda and eat more broccoli).

The next-most-common strategy was explanation, particularly explaining the rationale for a particular treatment. Done correctly, this can be very helpful, as it provides a logical hook for a patient to remember the treatment—"This medication lowers the acid level in the stomach, so may prevent reflux symptoms." But doctors easily get mired in excessively detailed, jargon-heavy explanations that end up burying the key take-home messages.

But not one of the doctors in this study used the strategies with the strongest track records: summarizing the information, suggesting that the patient take notes, and asking the patient to restate the key points.[7] Why don't doctors use these techniques? I thought about this after one particularly long clinic session. For every patient, there was just so much to convey that those techniques seemed overwhelming. Even for a patient with simple reflux like the actors in the study, I had to explain what the disease was, which foods could exacerbate it, how portion size and meal timing could affect the symptoms, what the medication options were, which red-flag signs to look out for. Plus there was the related advice that losing weight will help the reflux, and that involved a discussion about what the patient was currently eating, which food substitutions might be helpful, how exercise might fit in. And of course it is the exception not the rule that a patient comes with only one issue to discuss, so there were comparable discussions for each of the other concerns, plus a whole other discussion regarding general health-maintenance issues.

I'd tried to do a good job that day. I prioritized what was most important, tried to repeat those points for emphasis, even wrote the key points on paper for the patients (forcing myself to slow down to keep my penmanship passably legible is worse than the thumbscrew for me). But the thought of asking the patients to repeat back what we'd just reviewed—for each of the scores of topics we'd talked about—was simply too daunting. I could hardly stay afloat with all that I had to tell the patients and couldn't imagine how I could take more time to now ask them to tell me what they remembered. Even if I reminded myself that this would probably be a time-saver in the long run—if it enabled patients to do the things that would bring them relief—in the short run it felt like it might sink the ship entirely.

I reminded myself of my own experiment with letting patients talk uninterrupted at the beginning of each visit and how it hadn't eaten up as much time as I'd feared. Nevertheless, the fear of taking up more time with a teach-back session was enough to dissuade me. Indeed, in the study with actors, the doctors who used recall-enhancing techniques (even if they weren't using the best ones) took longer. Those who used the most ended up spending 50 percent more time than those who used the fewest.

Now I know that no one is suggesting doctors stop every thirty seconds to quiz patients on recall. We can certainly be selective and prioritize, but I am more struck by the paralyzing dread that this sort of thing engenders. We already have too much to cram into a short visit, with innumerable administrative mandates piled onto the clinical information, plus the ever-looming "quality metrics" that threaten to pounce on any shortfall. But the baby shouldn't be thrown out with the bathwater.

After reading all these studies, I thought long and hard about how I might incorporate some of this into my practice. Certainly the data on patients not knowing their doctors' names stuck with me. I make it a point now to repeat my name both at the beginning and end of a visit. And if we are in a situation with a whole circus of doctors involved, I try to slip in my name frequently, along with a reminder of what role I play in the cast of characters. (And if the patient *still* can't remember who I am, I fall back on my handy Oprah mnemonic. One of the first times in residency that I introduced myself as Dr. Ofri—pronounced OH-free—the patient, who was kind of a quirky fellow, replied, "Ofri, huh? Sorta like Oprah Winfrey." At the time, I thought it was just a random association from an idiosyncratic character. But throughout my years as a doctor, the Oprah Winfrey response has turned up with surprising regularity and from patients of all walks of life. I feel confident that it's because of our commensurate thespian skills, media-mogul acumen, and dashing diva aura, so I've found it convenient to summon up Oprah Winfrey whenever appellative clarification is needed.)

I also remind myself about the limited utility of constant repetition. I definitely want to emphasize key points, but I try to catch myself if I'm starting to harangue. Heidi E. Hamilton's research showing that patients overwhelmingly know the basic facts about their illnesses, like Tracey with her diabetes, has remained with me. Simply repeating "cut out the white rice, eat more vegetables" doesn't get anyone anywhere. When I find myself on the verge of trotting that phrase out again, I try to stop myself and instead ask, "What are the hardest challenges in dealing with diabetes?"

Nine times out of ten that question yields the most important kernel of the medical visit. If we are striving for efficiency—in the true sense of getting the most clinical meat within the short time allotted—that's the kind of question we should be asking up front.

Thus far, I've focused on how much patients remember of what doctors say. But I often wonder about the opposite: how much do doctors remember of what patients say? I hunted for research studies on that topic, and surprisingly (or unsurprisingly) could find none. There were no comparable studies testing what doctors remember of patients' names, diagnoses, or medical histories. I suppose this might seem like a ridiculous question because, after all, doctors have spent so many years memorizing for medical school that they must be good at remembering patients' information. Plus they have that handy medical chart with everything written down, right?

There were only small tangential studies about how much doctors recall of the information they read in medical journals (embarrassingly little)[8] or how well they remember clinical information from a fictionalized case study (full-fledged doctors do better than medical students),[9] but nothing with real patients.

There is one real-life experiment regarding physician memory that happens, unfortunately, a little too regularly. Electronic medical records have been revolutionary in many respects—a patient's chart can no longer be adrift in the cardiology clinic and a crucial X-ray can't be languishing in a surgeon's back pocket. However, by dint of being computerized, such information is susceptible to the same glitches as every other bit of computerized material. In the middle of writing your Tolstoy-worthy note about a patient with sixteen illnesses, the computer freezes, or the program crashes, or you inadvertently hit "escape" or "delete" at an inopportune moment, and all of your carefully wrought observations evaporate into the ether.

At least once a day, it seems, a medical student or intern will turn up, ashen-faced, stammering with incomprehensibility about the note they just lost, about all their efforts that just went up in smoke. Even the old hands at the hospital, who've learned the electronic landmines in trial-by-fire experience, are not immune. Recently I'd been writing a particularly complicated note about a patient with multiple chronic illnesses who was on more than a dozen medications and had numerous lab values out of whack, when I was interrupted by a phone call about an abnormal X-ray for a different patient. I had to open that patient's chart to untangle that issue. After sorting through that second patient's medical history and what to do about the X-ray, I went to close the second chart so I wouldn't commit the cardinal sin of mixing up two charts.

It took only a fraction of a second. Before I'd even released my finger from the mouse, I realized I'd closed the wrong tab. I kept my finger depressed on the mouse as long as I could, hoping that I could will that brief gesture into reverse, that I could telepathically conjure the information back onto the screen. When my irrational hopes could be sustained no longer and the boulder of despair had fully dropped anchor into my deepest bowels, I released my finger in agonizing slow motion.

I remained in vigorous denial for as long as I could, but finally my brain was forced to articulate what I already knew in my heart: I'd just lost everything. (And if you thought our vaunted electronic medical-record system would have something practical like auto-save to prevent such a mess, dream on!)

I'd lost all the information I'd taken down while the patient was in the room. I'd lost all the analysis I'd been writing after she'd left the room. (She was a new patient, so I'd done an extensive background history.) I'd lost all of the details of her prior medical evaluations. I'd lost my entire train of thought about her because I'd been forced to delve into another patient's medical history.

Honestly, I just wanted to cry. The injustice of it all punctured my day, and everything just deflated around me. I'd lost the mojo that was propelling me forward, and I could not imagine how I'd get through the rest of my patients. I'd entered that special circle of hell created by cocksure computer programmers whose systems can incinerate hours of work with breathtaking nanotech efficiency.

Even in my despair, though, I had to reluctantly acknowledge that my Dantean melodramatics were bordering on the histrionic. I'd lost a note, after all, not a patient. Despite all the effort that went into it, it was still just a bunch of writing. Life isn't fair, especially life mediated by technology—no matter what those singularity gurus preach. But as our middle school teachers have always patiently reminded us, everything is a teaching moment, and doctors losing their electronic notes is a fortuitous—if excruciating—natural experiment in measuring their recall of patients' words. Regrettably, this happens frequently enough to accumulate an informal mass of data.

Once I've chiseled myself up off the floor, the most expeditious thing to do is to simply grit my teeth and start writing from scratch, however repugnant it feels. Which is what I did for this patient. Trying my best to ignore both the buzz outside my office that continually reminds me that other patients are waiting and my own rising serum cortisol level that was inciting a faintly Pleistocene fight-or-flight response—is this @#$% software my personal mastodon?—I began pounding my fingers against the keyboard.

Whenever this happens, I am always amazed that I actually do remember many of the things I've written. Despite the overwrought fury and the metaphorical whacks against the side of the computer— sprinkled in with the occasional *actual* whacks that are embarrassingly satisfying—much of the information does come back.

What comes most effortlessly is the HPI, the history of the present illness. This is the information surrounding the primary reason the patient has decided to come to the doctor. In this case, I could easily remember that this patient had been treated for *H. pylori* gastritis a year ago, and she had continued the acid suppression treatment until the five refills of the prescription ran out. She didn't have time to get back to the doctor because she had a new job and was a single parent with a tenuous child-care arrangement. The symptoms gradually returned, though when I questioned her in detail about the specifics, the symptoms seemed much more like reflux than gastritis.

The other part I find easiest to remember is what's called the social history. I remembered that she was from the Pacific coast state of Guerrero—unlike most Mexicans in New York City, who come from the landlocked state of Puebla—and that she'd completed one year of university studying psychology. But then she and her husband decided it would be better for their daughter to be raised in America so they emigrated together. Unfortunately, their marriage didn't fare as well as their relocation and they separated soon after arriving in New York. She was working in a nail salon and studying to get a manicurist license. The hours were long and she usually arrived home after her daughter was already asleep. The daughter was recently diagnosed with mild autism and had started therapy in her kindergarten class.

But then I struggled with some of the other details. What year did she say her last Pap smear was? Was it her aunt who had colon cancer or her grandmother? Did she say she had a tetanus shot at another clinic, or was she talking about a PPD test for tuberculosis?

When I talk to the students and interns whom I've coached through similar electronic meltdowns, they have comparable experiences. The HPI and social history are the quickest to reformulate; other details can be sketchier. When I think about this from a literary perspective, the reason is obvious. The HPI is a story—there is a plot with twists and turns, challenges and conflicts. Stories are always easier to remember than lists of facts. And the social history is what writing teachers refer to as "fleshing out the character." Without the social history, the patient is just a stock character. A thirty-two-year-old woman with abdominal pain is as much a stock character in medicine as the tragic hero or the Southern belle or the wise old man are stock characters in fiction. These are stick figures until the writer fleshes them out to become Orpheus, Blanche DuBois, or Albus Dumbledore. They are now three-dimensional and realistic human beings who lodge themselves in our memories. And while the social history in the medical interview doesn't allow us the hundreds of pages that Tennessee Williams or J. K. Rowling can luxuriate in, it does permit us to get a fuller sense of our patients and some context of their lives. I may have forgotten what this patient's diastolic blood pressure was, but I could never forget the pained expression on her face when she spoke of how her job made her miss reading bedtime stories to her daughter each night and how she wasn't confident that the babysitter was reliably reading those stories to her daughter, who so needed the extra enrichment.

Of course the phone number of her next-of-kin contact that I'd responsibly typed into my note was completely lost, so I had to dash out to the waiting room to catch her before she left. And her answers to my detailed questions about diet—How many fruits and vegetables per week? How much soda? White bread or whole wheat bread?—were forever consigned to the electronic dustheap.

I'm impressed at what we are able to remember despite the acute misery of the circumstances. It may be the immediacy of the situation, like repeating a telephone number just long enough to memorize it in the short run, but I think it speaks more to which aspects of a human interaction—and a great novel—are most memorable: plot and character.

However, I'm well aware that this software-glitch experiment measures my memory only of what I *heard* the patient say. It doesn't tell me what I missed. It doesn't tell me what information sailed blithely past me as I was scribbling down answers from three questions ago. It doesn't tell me which facts I consciously or unconsciously chose to filter out. It doesn't tell me which underlying agendas remained undetected. It doesn't indicate what subtle body language sat unnoticed. It doesn't tell me if or how my internal biases altered, blocked, or otherwise transmogrified the information my patient was trying to convey to me.

Short of videotaping every doctor-patient interaction and then individually grilling the participants afterward, there isn't a foolproof way of precisely measuring what each party gleans from the conversational give-and-take. But there are a few simple things that doctors and patients can do. For the patient, there is always the standard advice to come to the doctor with a list of what you want to discuss. My only caveat is to be realistic with that list. Countless times I've had patients unfurl *Iliad*-length treatises, with scores of questions single-spaced, footnoted, annotated, and cross-referenced. So prioritizing the top two or three is crucial if you want to achieve anything beyond the superficial. At the other end of the visit, it really does pay for the patient to take a few notes. Jotting down—and verbally clarifying—the key points is invaluable.

For the doctor, briefly summarizing what the patient has said—the technique least used in the study with actors but the most effective—can work without taking as much time as we fear. "Let me see if I've got this right" is a simple way to initiate a brief restatement of the facts. Not only does this serve as a great way to get the facts straight, but it's also a solid indicator to the patient that you are actually listening. Knowing that you are being heard is the building block of trust and empathy,[10] something Corine Jansen demonstrated over and over. For the doctors who feel this might take too much time, I assure you this is money in the bank. It will repay itself in terms of more accurate information upon which to make a diagnosis, enhanced trust from your patient, and just a much more enjoyable experience for the fifteen minutes—and hopefully fifteen years—that follow. Plus you are probably much less likely to get sued, but more on that in the next chapter.

And then at the end of the visit, even though you are afraid of opening a Pandora's box and running even later than you already are, ask, "Is there anything that we missed?" While I do not have any data to back this up, my sense is that the very act of asking this question makes the patient *less* likely to bring up anything else. For most patients, knowing that the door is open to ask another question in the future allays the anxiety of trying to cram everything into one visit. And for the rare patient who follows the *Iliad*-length HPI with an *Odyssey*-like response to that final question, you are well within your constitutional rights to suggest that this would make an excellent basis for your next visit together.

CHAPTER 10

Do No Harm

Patients typically sue because they are dissatisfied with the outcome of their medical care. Sometimes the reasons are obvious, such as a surgeon operating on the wrong leg. Sometimes it is outright negligence, such as a doctor not prescribing antibiotics when they were clearly needed. Sometimes the case is coaxed forth by the stereotypical ambulance-chasing lawyer. Often it is simply a bad medical outcome, without any obvious fault or flaw, but that is enough to get the malpractice ball rolling.

But the underlying commonality is almost always a breakdown in doctor-patient communication. A group of researchers analyzed four thousand pages of depositions filed by patients and noted "problematic relationship issues" in almost three-quarters of the cases.[1] When they dissected the depositions in more detail, three communication shortcomings arose repeatedly: doctors did not deliver information well, doctors didn't take patients' viewpoints seriously, and doctors didn't understand their patients' perspectives. (The fourth common theme in these depositions was that many patients felt abandoned by their doctors during their medical care. I suppose one could consider this a form of communications breakdown—a particularly heinous one—but I'll leave it aside for now.)

It should come as no surprise that doctors and patients see things quite differently when it comes to malpractice. In one large survey of doctors and patients who'd ever been involved in lawsuits,[2]

97 percent of patients cited physician negligence as their reason for suing. Of doctors who had been involved in lawsuits, a mere 10 percent felt negligence had occurred. By comparison, doctors who had never been sued estimated that negligence occurred in about 50 percent of malpractice cases.

More than three-quarters of doctors, regardless of whether they'd been sued, felt that financial motivation was a primary reason for malpractice suits. Only a fifth of patients agreed with that statement. Doctors and patients also had very different takes on the doctor-patient relationship. The vast majority of doctors were quite confident that they were offering an honest, open relationship, but fewer than half of patients reported experiencing it that way.

In fact, there was only one thing in the entire survey that the doctors and the patients agreed upon: two-thirds of both groups felt that improving doctor-patient communication would decrease lawsuits.

But is that true? Does better communication between doctors and patients make malpractice suits less likely? Using Debra Roter's RIAS analysis system, linguistics researchers tried to answer this question by examining in depth ten office visits for each of 124 doctors.[3] Roughly half the doctors were primary-care doctors (general internists and family doctors). The other half were orthopedic surgeons. They analyzed how these doctors spoke and interacted with their patients to see if any particular behavior could predict which were the doctors who had been sued (based on insurance company records).

Among the primary-care doctors, length of visit was the strongest predictor. Those who had never been sued spent 20 percent more time with their patients. Other notable differences were that doctors who had never been sued spent more time outlining what the patient might expect—both for the clinical condition and for the logistics of the medical evaluation. They also encouraged the patient to talk and frequently asked the patients' opinions. They checked in to see if the patients understood what was going on. There was also more laughter and humor in these visits.

It can't necessarily be said that these behaviors *prevented* lawsuits. Things could work in the reverse—doctors devastated by lawsuits might be more tight-lipped in conversation, more wary of extending conversation beyond the necessary (certainly studies have consistently shown that doctors experience much less joy in medicine after a lawsuit). But thinking back to the analysis of the depositions filed by patients, the prime frustrations were that they were not being heard and that things were not communicated clearly to them. So these observations about the primary-care doctors who were never sued versus those who had been sued make sense. And from an economic standpoint regarding malpractice prevention, a few more minutes talking is a lot cheaper than the billions of dollars spent annually on defensive medicine.

Interestingly, among the orthopedic surgeons, there weren't major differences in communication styles between those who'd been sued and those who hadn't. However, another study by the same research group focused specifically on tone of voice in surgeons.[4] Ten-second clips of the surgeon speaking, taken from the first and last minute of the visit, were analyzed for tone. The tone could be rated from one to seven for each of the following qualities: warm, concerned, interested, satisfied, genuine, professional, competent, sympathetic, anxious, hostile, and dominant. Then, using these ratings, the researchers tried to see which qualities of voice tone could predict which surgeons had been sued in the past. Unsurprisingly, perhaps, it turned out that surgeons who rated highest on the dominant scale and lowest on the concern and warmth scales were those who were most likely to have been sued.

Again, it's hard to dissect out the cause and effect. Patients may be less likely to sue doctors who are more open to hearing their views, who help them know what to expect, and who have a less overbearing way of speaking. Or, it might be that doctors with those traits are better clinicians and make fewer errors. A third possibility is that none of these traits affects the risk of lawsuit, and it's just that doctors who have been sued end up less sympathetic, more dominant, and less likely to engage with patients. It's impossible to know which way the causality runs.

Nevertheless, these studies suggest some good guidelines for doctors: don't be too overbearing, get a sense of the patient's perspective, and do your best to let patients know what to expect, including the possible bad outcomes.

Malpractice suits, of course, are only the tip of the iceberg when it comes to medical care that doesn't turn out the way all parties hope. The scope of medical malfeasance is a far more sprawling field: errors, complications, misdiagnoses, and untoward outcomes. This broader field is more challenging to study because there aren't clear registries of data, as there are for malpractice suits. But how doctors and patients communicate in all of these circumstances is critically important.

An interesting story about communication in this realm took place a few years ago at a sleepy VA hospital in Lexington, Kentucky. Steve Kraman is a pulmonologist with a specialty in critical-care medicine, and in 1986 he became the chief of staff at the Lexington VA. The hospital had just lost two bruising malpractice suits that cost it $1.5 million plus incalculable effort and pain. Kraman and the hospital's chief attorney, Ginny Hamm, were put in charge of a risk management program designed to learn about errors early on, before they snowballed into malpractice suits. The committee hung out their shingle and let it be known that they wanted to be informed of any medical errors that occurred in the hospital.

The silence was deafening—and unsurprising.

"Nobody came forward with errors," said Kraman, a slim, bespectacled physician with a trim mustache and beard, "so we had to do a bit of snooping." And it didn't take long to uncover a smoking gun.

An alcoholic woman, admitted with dehydration and electrolyte depletion, had died on a recent night in the hospital. The death was attributed to severe malnutrition brought about by decades of alcohol use and had aroused no suspicions at the time. During the treatment course the patient had been given fluids, along with intravenous potassium to correct a dangerously low potassium level. The resident physician had ordered blood tests that afternoon to recheck the patient's potassium level, with a plan to decide whether the potassium drip needed to be continued or stopped. The labs were drawn but the resident became swamped with work and forgot to check them. The potassium continued to drip methodically into the patient's veins.

For entirely different reasons—the patient had complained of palpitations—a Holter monitor happened to be hooked up to the patient. Holter monitors are little boxes that hang around a patient's neck, recording the EKG for a full day or more. These are usually given to outpatients, so there's no visible monitor on the outside; it's just a box that contains the data. When the patient was discovered dead, the Holter monitor was shoved aside as weightier things were attended to.

But the Holter monitor wended its way back to the cardiology lab, and in due time the contents of the device were downloaded. The pages and pages of printout eventually made their way to the top of a staff cardiologist's pile.

The electrical output of the heart—the EKG—is a delicate, squiggling affair, with waves, peaks, and valleys corresponding to the electrical signaling during the cardiac cycle. The QRS complex is a spike that corresponds to the contraction of the ventricles. The T-wave, a semicircular hump toward the end of the cycle, indicates relaxation. Potassium is critically involved in the electrical conduction of heart cells, so EKG morphology can be a mirror of potassium levels in the blood.

What the cardiologist saw in the Holter reading was a textbook progression of rising potassium levels. First, the smooth T-waves grew peaked. Then the spikes of the QRS complex widened. Then all the spikes and waves began to soften, jellylike, and drift apart from one another, degenerating into an amorphous sine-wave slush. And finally it all collapsed into what doctors charitably call asystole, the featureless horizon of flatline that stretches out to a desolate eternity.

This is not what cardiologists typically view on routine outpatient Holter reports, and one can imagine the gripping fear in the heart of this one as the inexorable march toward death was documented in excruciatingly accurate detail. This patient clearly had died of a hyperkalemic (high-potassium) cardiac arrest, though no one had known it at the time.

When Kraman—a critical-care specialist—saw the Holter, he knew before he'd even exhaled a single breath that the VA had a wrongful death on its hands. You couldn't have evidence any more incriminating than this minute-to-minute, time-stamped Holter readout. But what to do with this information? The patient's family had taken her body; the funeral had already occurred. There had been no concerns at the time about the death; both the family and the doctors had accepted the readily available explanation that the patient had died of her severe alcoholism. The desire to let sleeping dogs lie could not be denied.

But there was no question in Kraman's mind about what to do. The hospital called the family, told them that some new information had come to light about their loved one's death, and that the hospital staff would like to talk with them. Oh, and they should bring a lawyer.

"We never want to reveal what happened during the initial phone call," Kraman says, "but we do want to indicate its seriousness so that the family will definitely show up. Telling them to bring a lawyer usually accomplishes that."

The risk management staff met with the family and explained that they had strong evidence that a medical error had been made and that the hospital was directly responsible for the death. "When we told them," Kraman recalled, "the family was certainly shocked, but it was their attorney whose jaw dropped. He could not believe we were voluntarily disclosing this information." The hospital took responsibility for the death, offered a settlement, and within a few weeks there was an agreement.

The fact that a lawsuit had been averted—one the hospital surely would have lost—became the impetus for a new hospital policy mandating full disclosure. The goal was that all errors would be fully and promptly disclosed to the patient or family—most certainly not the standard way most doctors communicated errors to patients.

Every single untoward incident had to be reported. A peer review committee would do an evaluation to decide if there actually was an error. For example, if a patient died of pneumonia despite being given three different antibiotics but the antibiotics had all been appropriate choices, this would not be considered an error. But if a true error were uncovered, the disclosure gears would grind forward. All medical errors—including invisible ones and near misses—would be proactively disclosed to the patients and their families. Sleeping dogs would not be allowed to lie.

Telling patients the truth about errors, even about near misses, is, of course, the right thing to do. Every doctor would say that this is the ethically correct course of action. But I know from brutal experience that this is far from easy.

It was during a long night on call—we were probably up to our eighth or ninth admission that day, but my intern and I had long since given up counting. I was midway through my medical residency at Bellevue and was already a seasoned survivalist; you had to be, otherwise you'd drown in the overwhelming pummel of admissions that streamed in from the ER, day and night.

This admission was a classic eye-roller: a nursing home patient with dementia, sent to our hospital for altered mental status. When you were juggling patients with bleeding ulcers, acute heart failure, fulminant septicemia, raging diabetic infections, and multidrug overdoses, it was hard to get worked up about a demented nonagenarian who someone thought was looking perhaps a wee bit more demented that day. The patient was totally stable, I was told—labs fine, radiology fine.

The trick to surviving on call was to "turf" as quickly and as aggressively as possible. Anyone you could possibly turf to another service—surgery, rehab, psych—was one less on your ever-expanding list. This patient was a perfect candidate for the so-called intermediate-care unit, which was a back corner of the hospital that functioned as a holding station for patients with no active medical issues, patients just awaiting discharge arrangements.

But the covering doc left at 5 p.m., so we'd have to work quickly—assemble the labs, head CT, chest X-ray. Once we'd ruled out any treatable medical explanation for the altered mental status, we could safely turf the patient. It was 4:45 p.m., and I scanned through the labs as I dialed the covering doctor. I quickly ran down the case to her: demented patient, totally stable, labs fine, radiology fine, just needs to get back to his nursing home.

I remember the doctor's voice so clearly over the phone. She had an Indian lilt to her voice, and she asked me, "You're sure the labs and scans are normal?" Yes, yes, yes, I pressed her. Totally stable. Everything is fine.

The doctor hesitated; taking a patient so near to closing time wasn't ideal. I reassured her that the patient was completely stable, that there was no work for her to do, and eventually she relented. The intern and I high-fived each other and then bolted to the ER for the rest of the night, sifting through the admissions that had piled up. There were patients with cellulitis, emphysema, unstable angina, and pancreatitis. Illness never seemed to end, especially during those long nights on call.

It wasn't until early the next afternoon that I learned that my "totally stable" patient had spent the night in the operating room. It turned out he actually had an intracranial hemorrhage—he was bleeding into his brain. *That's* why his mental status was altered. The covering doctor didn't mince words when she told me how she'd been paged during the night by the radiologist who saw the bleed on the head CT. The patient was whisked out by the neurosurgeons for emergency surgery to drain the blood inside his skull.

My body felt like it was turning to stone as all my metabolic processes ground to a halt. An intracranial bleed? A hemorrhage into the brain? You couldn't get much worse than missing an intracranial bleed. But I had. I had failed to check the head CT before jettisoning the patient. Someone had said "radiology fine" and I hadn't looked at the actual scan myself, as I knew I should have.

The covering doctor stormed away before I could even open my mouth, which was just as well because I was incapable of speech. If I could have willed myself to melt away on the spot, to melt myself out of existence—I would have.

In cerebral academic analysis, this incident would be classified as a near miss because the patient's medical care ultimately proceeded correctly. The multiple layers of care in the hospital ensured that the intracranial bleed was correctly diagnosed and treated. Appropriate medical care had not been impacted, or even delayed really, by my oversight.

But I had still made the error. What if I had prescribed a medication such as aspirin that could have furthered the bleeding? What if it had been earlier in the day and I'd sent the patient back to the nursing home in an ambulette that lacked resuscitation equipment? What if the radiologist hadn't read the scan until the next day? The "what-ifs" were endless, and endlessly tormenting. My error could easily have led to a fatal outcome. It was nothing but sheer luck that saved the patient from my bungling error.

I was horrified at myself for not performing due diligence for my patient, mortified that I had relied on a verbal report rather than taking the time to examine the CT scan myself. The shame was blistering and all encompassing. No matter how I rationalized to myself that the patient was unharmed and that the system of checks and balances in the hospital had functioned appropriately, I was still faced with the unvarnished truth: I had committed a life-threatening medical error.

I was so ashamed that I didn't tell anyone about my lapse—not that day and not ever after. I didn't tell my intern. I didn't tell my attending. And I certainly couldn't fathom dragging my sorry self into the patient's room to come clean. I would sooner knock back a mug of the muck-strewn waters of the East River just outside the hospital than face the patient with my inexcusable oversight. All I wanted to do was barricade myself into a broom closet and mope among the cleaning supplies.

It is precisely for this emotional reason that Kraman's team would not have the "offending" physician present at the family meeting. "The first ten minutes can be a bit hot," he said, and this struck me as an affable but staggering understatement. "There can be accusations, anger." If the doctor got defensive it could defeat the whole purpose of the meeting.

Carol Liebman disagrees with this. Liebman is a clinical professor of law at Columbia University who has been interested in medical mediation as a way to improve patient safety and possibly—as a byproduct—minimize lawsuits. Her group decided to offer free mediation services to hospitals in exchange for being able to study the process and interview the participants.[5] The goal was to figure out how communication and mediation could both shorten the process and ease the arduousness that typically attends medical errors.

The parties to a medical error—patients, families, doctors, administrators, lawyers—typically disagree on the key elements of a case, but the one thing they *do* agree on is that the current malpractice process is inefficient, costly, and just plain dreadful. Like a Band-Aid being haltingly peeled off, the misery seems designed to be meted out in excruciating slow motion. No one ends up pleased, even those who "win" the case. When you talk to people who have prevailed in a malpractice case, they will rarely speak of joy or even satisfaction at winning. It's more like relief that a marathon of emotional exhaustion has finally ceased. Could mediation offer something better than that protracted agony?

Liebman described a case to me that centered on the placement of a central line. When central lines are placed in either the subclavian or jugular vein, there is always the risk of puncturing the top margins of the lungs, which are parked amid these prominent vessels. A pneumothorax, as it's called, is a known complication of central lines, though thankfully not common. And if it *does* happen, the pneumothorax is usually minuscule. A tiny sliver of lung deflates, and then generally reinflates on its own with no notable consequences. But if the pneumothorax is massive—which is extremely rare from a central line, more likely from a motor vehicle accident—enough oxygen supply can be cut off to lead to cardiovascular collapse.

In this case, a patient was getting a subclavian line from a resident physician. Stuart Benson suffered from emphysema, which eats away at the taut orderly air sacs of the lungs, leaving the organs filled with the equivalent of unkempt, oversized, saggy balloons. Emphysematous lungs lack the firm recoil of healthy lungs and possess little physiologic reserve.

Tragically, the tip of the resident's needle punctured Mr. Benson's fragile lung, which promptly deflated. The massive pneumothorax acutely sapped his body of oxygen and his heart went into cardiac arrest. Mr. Benson did not survive.

The resident called Mrs. Benson at home and told her to come to the hospital immediately, though he didn't give her the reason. When she arrived, the attending physician met her outside her husband's room. The attending informed Mrs. Benson of her husband's untimely death. After that, though, Mrs. Benson was left in the hallway while the medical team tended to all the things that medical teams attend to after a patient has died. The staff eventually dispersed, the communications petered out, and Mrs. Benson was left stranded in the hallway, literally and figuratively.

That feeling of being stranded in the hallway is regrettably common and is often the prime motivation behind lawsuits. I've never met Mrs. Benson, but I can only imagine the enormity of what she was facing. Losing a spouse is already one of life's most harrowing moments. Grief is emotion enough to consume a person, but to then have anger elbow in on that grief can be corrosive. There is anger at being abandoned by the doctors, anger at not knowing how or why her husband died, anger at having her private grief be contaminated by this unwanted bitterness. I imagine that filing a lawsuit was probably the last thing she'd want to do while mourning the death of her life partner. That she did is a testament to how potent the anger in such situations can be and how long it can fester.

Because of the drawn-out pace of such proceedings, it was nearly a year after Mr. Benson's death when all the parties finally met in one room. "When the hospital team arrived at the mediation," Liebman told me, "the widow's face fell when she saw that the doctor who'd placed the central line wasn't there." From Mrs. Benson's perspective, the hospital's taking of responsibility was hollow if the person who'd actually caused the error wasn't part of the human equation.

The mediation process allowed Mrs. Benson to ask questions about the central line and why a resident physician was doing the procedure. It allowed her to express her anger and frustration at how she had been treated. But the lack of communication with the doctor directly responsible was undermining the credibility needed for mediation to work. Trust was fast eroding and it seemed a lawsuit might be inevitable.

At the second mediation session, however, the chief of medicine had something to add. He mentioned that he had seen the resident that morning and had asked him if he remembered the patient—it had been almost a year since the incident, after all. The physician's response was both incredulous and pained. "*Remember* him? I think of him every single day. I grieve for him every day." When this quote was relayed to the widow, the atmosphere changed immediately. Even though the doctor was not present, his emotions—particularly his remorse, his pain, and the enduring ramifications—restored an important degree of humanity to the process, and the widow was more open to what the team had to say. The sides agreed to a fair settlement and a protracted, painful, adversarial fight was averted. There was a financial payment but also a commitment from the hospital to improve its care—something that is a critical ingredient in responding to the pain experienced by families. A safety checklist for central lines was instituted. The hospital also ramped up its training for the staff on how to communicate with family members in the event of a death, so that no one would be left standing in the hallway.

Liebman feels it is critically important for the person who made the error to personally acknowledge the error, take responsibility, and, most critically, apologize. Even when there isn't a clear-cut cause—as there was in the case of the central line—the spoken words of acknowledgment and apology are critical. Nothing can move forward without them.

I agree with her but I also know how arduous this can be. After I had missed that intracranial bleed I was so overcome with shame that I didn't have the inner resources to tell even my supervising attending, let alone tell the patient. My error took place before the widespread acceptance of full disclosure, but I knew coming clean was the ethically correct thing to do. I had no doubts about that. Nevertheless, I simply couldn't. It's true that the atmosphere of medical training at the time wasn't conducive to such admissions, but I couldn't blame it wholly on that. My resistance was internal.

Looking back now, I see the missed opportunities so clearly and so poignantly. Had I felt comfortable enough to tell my attending on that morning, she could have helped me understand how the error occurred and how to prevent it in the future. Even more powerfully, she could have taken our team to the bedside and modeled how a doctor might speak to a patient about an error. So much of what we learn in medical training is promptly forgotten, but this is the type of teaching moment that resonates forever.

Apart from the error itself and the ramifications for the patient and family, there is also the devastating effect on the person who made the error. As a barely-out-of-the-gates doctor, my missing the intracranial bleed was cataclysmic. Until that moment I'd thought I was a reasonably good doctor—no worse or no better than my colleagues—but in a split second that entire persona came shattering down. It wasn't just that I had made an error; it was that my being a doctor was an error. I felt like such a crashing disappointment to my profession that the only prudent course would be to take down my shingle, such as it was, and barricade myself at a desk job alphabetizing insurance forms, selflessly sparing future innocents my shabby medical ministering.

Sacrificing my medical career—as dramatic and tempting as it felt—was simply not an option, though. Calling in sick for even a single day was practically verboten, because everyone else had to shoulder your work. If you had the audacity and selfishness to quit outright, your fellow residents would probably flay you before your grubby white coat even landed in the laundry bin. The only acceptable reasons to abandon ship were permanent coma, cardiac arrest, or possibly a full-body cast, but even that was dubious.

Unable to commit my noble hari-kari, I simply plowed on. I showed up every day at 7 a.m., rounded on my patients, wrote in the charts, attended noon conferences, but I was numb, paralyzed by an all-consuming shame. Had I been able to tell my attending about my error, maybe she could have eased the dreadfulness of the weeks that followed. I say this with empathy not only for my younger self, but also for the patients I cared for in those weeks. With my soul in a fog and my brain in permanent low gear, who knows how many little things I missed—the slightly depressed bicarb level, the subtle signs of a wound infection, the incrementally prolonged QT interval on an EKG. I'm certain there was a trail of errors in the wake of my missing that intracranial bleed—many of which could have been avoided if I'd been able to speak openly about what had happened. The shame burrowed so deep and with such tenacity that it took me a full twenty years to finally be able to speak of that moment.

Steve Kraman, who is now a professor of medicine at the University of Kentucky, is convinced that the full-disclosure experience can help dissolve the poisonous culture that inhibits people from doing the right thing. "Mostly these are honest mistakes by good people," he told me, and I found myself grateful for the forgiveness and optimism of those words, even these many years after my error. "Usually they were overworked, or their attention wavered for just a moment." From the way he described it, I could see how the disclosure-and-restitution process could offer some balm for the person who'd made the error. And, it turned out, lawsuits were indeed fewer.[6]

The decrease in lawsuits and overall financial payout at the VA garnered a significant amount of media attention. Other hospitals found similar results after implementing comparable programs.[7] In fact, an entire organization—Sorry Works!—was formed to promulgate this full-disclosure-and-restitution policy. A self-described "middle ground" for doctors, patients, insurers, lawyers, and hospitals, Sorry Works! is an advocacy group for this new way of thinking. Its website offers testimonials from people for whom an apology averted a lawsuit, and others for whom an apology never materialized and led to bitter litigation.

In reading the plethora of news articles on their website, I was struck by the cheerfully righteous tone as they exclaimed over the counterintuitive conclusion that hospitals have been saving money by full disclosure of error. This is almost divine justice: virtue is rewarded, good guys finish first, doing the right thing brings accolades and cost-savings . . . just like your mother always promised.

What a wonderful conclusion: full disclosure and an apology make a patient less likely to sue. I am wholly supportive of this important work. Lowering the number of lawsuits is salutary for every party involved: doctors, patients, administrators, insurers (well, maybe not for the malpractice lawyers. . .). However, it doesn't bring the risk to zero. From the hospital's perspective, decreasing lawsuits from four per year to one per year is a vast improvement. But for the one doctor who is still sued, that 75 percent decrease is meaningless. For that one doctor, it is a 100 percent life-altering experience, almost always devastating.

The hospital and the individual physician have very different agendas when it comes to disclosing errors and apologizing, and they also have fundamentally different things at stake. A hospital is rarely destroyed by a single malpractice suit, but an individual physician surely can be. The emotional and financial toll can permanently scorch a doctor's life—even if the doctor is acquitted.

The shame of error, with its attendant loss of sense of self, is an individual, human trait. Organizations rarely suffer from shame. After the money is forked over and the publicity dies down, hospitals continue on as they always have. Not so for the individual physician or the nurse; the emotional ravage tunnels deep into the soul. A veteran ICU nurse in Seattle committed suicide after her error led to the death of an eight-month-old baby.[8]

In the end, though, even if the data convincingly prove that the sophisticated communication skills of disclosure and apology lead to fewer lawsuits, I believe the desired culture of openness will come about only when we address the issue of shame. No matter how rational we doctors claim to be, the fragility of the human heart will override hard data, ethics, and even laws.

When thinking about how to improve communication between doctors and patients regarding medical error, it's clear we have to attend to the emotions on both sides. But doctors and patients have different stakes and expectations in that inevitable conversation. Patients overwhelmingly say they want as much information as possible. They want to know about any and all errors that may have occurred, even the minor ones. When researchers interviewed patients about this, there was absolute unanimity that *all* information should be disclosed.[9]

Physicians interviewed in the same study agreed with the patients, at least in theory. In practice, however, they were more circumspect. Doctors worried a lot about medical error and agreed that errors needed to be disclosed, but they felt strongly that they had to "choose their words carefully." They agreed they needed to be honest and accurate but they also felt the need to portray the events in the least negative way possible. The fear of a lawsuit is so pervasive that doctors worry any admission of error is tantamount to handing your head to a lawyer on a stainless steel surgical tray.

Researchers in this particular study conducted in-depth focus groups with doctors and patients in the same room. For half the session, the doctors sat in an inner circle discussing the issues while the patients observed from an outer circle. The situation was reversed for the second half of the session. This arrangement led to some of the most interesting observations of the study.

Patients were quite surprised to hear how deeply doctors were upset by errors they'd made. Most had assumed that like illness and death, errors and bad outcomes were all in a day's work for doctors. The patients were astonished by the depth and duration of anguish that doctors experienced. One patient remarked, "I was really surprised to hear the doctors talk like that. I saw a lot more caring than I expected. . . . You know, most of the time when you see the doctor you don't get their feelings. Yeah, I was surprised."

When the circles were reversed, doctors were surprised to learn that assigning blame was by no means the top priority for patients. As with Mrs. Benson, the primary goal was to obtain information. A close second was to know that the doctors and the hospital accepted responsibility and learned from the mistake. Blame was not the focus. This would support the experiences of the Lexington VA and the Sorry Works! group: acknowledgment, meaningful apology, and concrete actions to improve things go a long way toward repairing the harm. In fact, these probably accomplish more than a lawsuit, which is as bruising for the patient as for the doctor.

When it comes to acknowledging and apologizing, what seems to matter is the patient's perception of what the doctor says, even more than the actual words.[10] A group of researchers in Baltimore showed videos of three medical-error enactments to a group of volunteers. The simulated errors included a delay in noticing a mammogram report that indicated a possible cancer, a chemotherapy error in which the dose was ten-fold too high, and a patient who suffered a cardiac arrest after a surgeon was slow to answer a page.

For each medical error scenario, there were several versions of the video so that the researchers could vary whether or not the doctor accepted responsibility and whether or not the doctor apologized. Furthermore, there were two versions of the apology—one in which the doctor gave a generic apology ("I'm sorry that things turned out badly") and one that included a more directly personal apology ("I'm sorry that I gave the wrong dosage of chemotherapy").

As expected, the viewers gave higher ratings to the doctors who accepted responsibility and made a personal apology. But the fascinating finding was that what seemed to matter most was whether the viewer *perceived* these things as having occurred. If he or she perceived that the doctor made a personal apology (even if the video was scripted to be a nonspecific apology), then the viewer rated the doctor as more trustworthy.

Making an apology, though, is never easy. Acknowledging that you've made a mistake or fallen short can be painful, especially for doctors. I recently had this experience with a healthy, middle-aged, white woman whom I'd seen just once before, a year earlier, for a routine checkup. I ushered Kim Fuller into my office with a smile, prepared for another straightforward visit. "What can I help you with today?" I asked, as I always do to start a visit.

She stared stonily at the wall in front of her as my question hung, too long, in the air. "I almost didn't come back today," she finally said. "I was ready to choose another doctor but I decided to give you a second chance."

There was a reflexive start in my chest from her unexpectedly harsh reply but I held my composure. I quickly scanned the chart from our last visit to see if there had been anything we'd disagreed about or any unresolved issues. But no, it had been a routine checkup. Nothing beyond standard health screening issues and a run-of-the-mill tension headache.

"Someone had said you were a good doctor," Ms. Fuller said derisively, still addressing the wall, "but I was not impressed. My previous doctor, even though he was just a resident in training, was much better than you."

That certainly stung. And I still had no idea what had occurred between us to inspire her vitriol, so I endeavored to stay quiet, to simply listen. "But he graduated," she continued, "and now I'm stuck with you." She folded her arms across her chest, pursed her lips, and then was silent.

I sat there trying to figure out the best way to approach this situation. Should I apologize even though I didn't know what I'd done? Should I admit ignorance and ask directly what the transgression had been? Should I pretend to remember and try to craft a passable apology? I glanced again at the chart to find some clue, any clue, as to what I might have done to upset this patient so much. But I couldn't find a hint of anything. I decided honesty was better than faking it. I kept my voice as low key as possible and said, "I'm so sorry if there was something that upset you. I'm trying to recall—"

"You don't remember?" she snapped. "It figures!"

Now I was scraping desperately around in my mind. What had I done? Making a patient livid isn't something you typically forget but I couldn't come up with anything for Ms. Fuller. I realized I was going to have to offer blanket contrition, both for whatever had transpired between us and for my inability to remember it.

"I apologize," I said, as genuinely as I could, "but I honestly don't recall what happened. Could you tell me?"

Ms. Fuller looked at me for the first time, her eyes taut and icy. The pause before she spoke uncoiled tortuously, serrated with resentment. "You didn't do a physical exam. All you did was talk to me! That's all. My old doctor *always* did a physical exam but you didn't even bother."

My jaw actually dropped when she said that. I'd forgotten to do the physical exam? That was a biggie! How could I have done that?

As an internist, I'm well aware of the limits of the modern physical exam. For most medical ailments, nearly all the crucial diagnostic information is gathered in the history, in the conversation between doctor and patient. The physical exam serves mainly to confirm the diagnosis but it nevertheless remains an important part of the interaction between doctor and patient.

I felt like a complete idiot. Looking back at my notes, I honestly couldn't tell if I had been running late that day, or was distracted, or simply had a momentary lapse. Part of me wanted to defend the academic truth that the physical exam wasn't really necessary in a healthy patient with no symptoms other than a mild tension headache. I wanted to point out that the risk of a false positive result—finding something you think is abnormal but really isn't—outweighed any benefits by a long shot, and that by this reasoning you could say a physical exam in a healthy patient like her was more likely to cause harm than offer benefit. Maybe I'd actually given her *better* medical care by not doing the physical exam. But I knew that wouldn't go over well. And the unvarnished truth was that I'd neglected a standard part of the medical visit and the patient was appropriately calling me on it. There was really only one option for me.

"I am truly sorry," I said to her. "I honestly have no idea why I didn't do a physical exam that day. I really don't." I placed my hands down on the desk between us. "I can only offer you an apology, both for my shortcoming that day and for the bad feeling that it left you with."

Ms. Fuller gave a brief nod of acknowledgment and the muscles of her face softened by a few degrees. Our gazes simultaneously traveled to the exam table and then back to each other, questioning. "It's up to you," I said, hesitantly. "I would completely understand if you would feel more comfortable with a new doctor."

She shrugged. "Like I said, I'm willing to give you a second chance."

It was an awkward physical exam, no doubt for both of us. I felt like I was being given a test but appreciated the opportunity to face up to a mistake and work through it, however uncomfortable the experience.

Though "objective" measures of "quality" abound in medicine these days, getting meaningful feedback is actually quite rare. Getting it directly from a patient, rather than on a spreadsheet from an institution—or in a subpoena from a court—is rarer still. And even though it's never pleasant to be reminded of your shortcomings, I ultimately felt quite lucky that this patient had the grit to come back and tell me directly. She could just as easily have moved on to another doctor, and I never would have known.

It makes me wonder how many other times I have disappointed a patient but been completely unaware. I'm sure the number is larger than I'd care to acknowledge, and probably rising as time pressures and documentation requirements mount.

I thanked Ms. Fuller for giving me a second chance and we parted reasonably cordially. But I'll have to wait a year until her next annual visit to see if I passed the test.

CHAPTER 11

What Lies Beneath

200/110!!! The blood-pressure reading was printed in blaring red ink at the top of Bernice Ruger's chart. The medical assistant had evidently been concerned that I might miss the sky-high reading, so had added three exclamation points for emphasis. Mrs. Ruger was a new patient, an eighty-one-year-old white woman whom I'd never met before, but I could tell we'd be spending a lot of time talking about hypertension and how it causes strokes and heart attacks and other *horribilia*. Her chart listed at least three blood pressure pills, which, from the numbers, I assumed she wasn't taking, so I steeled myself for a talk about medication adherence as well.

Mrs. Ruger strode into my room like a hurricane, carrying a cane that didn't touch the ground once. She sat herself in the chair and leaned in so close to me that I could see the crackles in her pink lipstick where it fell outside the lines of her lips. Colossal red-framed eyeglasses dominated the geography of her face, leaving little territory that wasn't refracted by the powerful corrective lenses.

"I can't take any of your pills," she rasped at me before I could even introduce myself, her voice mottled by decades of cigarettes. "They make me sick." She paused. "Sick!!"

I eyed Mrs. Ruger, trying to figure out the best approach to her forceful opening gambit, but she didn't give me a chance to talk.

"That fosinopril? It made me sick! That water pill? It made me sick! That amlodipine? Sick! They all made me sick! I can't take a single one of them." She rattled off a panoply of symptoms: muscle spasms, nausea, headache, skin irritation, blurry vision, twitching tongue, stuffy nose, ringing in her ears, tingling in her chest, strange tastes in her mouth. With each emphatic pronouncement, her helmet of teased blond hair bobbed forcefully ever closer to my face, issuing wafts of hairspray smell. Mrs. Ruger listed six more medications that made her sick, then sat her petite, grandmotherly body back in her chair and clamped her hands decisively over her cane handle.

The prosecution had clearly rested its case.

Medicine is a science—I get that. Elucidating pathophysiology and evaluating evidence from clinical trials are the scientific underpinnings of what we doctors do. But there are days when medicine feels much more like an improvisation, something akin to what Richard Street, the professor of communications at Texas A&M, had suggested. You are thrown on stage with a complete stranger who can toss out an opening maneuver on any topic, in any key, in any language, from any one of a million locations beyond left field, and you need to step right in, without any hesitation, as if you had studied that exact script only moments before and were just waiting for that specific cue to begin.

In truth, the openings of most patient encounters fall into a very manageable number of varieties, and once you practice medicine long enough, you are in fact able to step right into most of them without missing a beat. But Mrs. Ruger was a reminder that exceptions aren't that rare and that the variety is infinite.

The initial communication between doctor and patient sets the tone for the rest of visit. Indeed it can set the tone for the rest of the doctor-patient relationship over years. Thus, whenever I'm presented with a patient who pitches forward so forcefully, I try to take a moment to think before I speak. What could the underlying agenda be? Years of working with patients (and plenty of bruising experiences with teenagers) has taught me that what's initially said is often completely unrelated to what the real issue is.

I gazed at Mrs. Ruger, whose posture had assumed a triumphant air. Hardly three minutes had elapsed and she'd already grabbed the visit by the reins and thrown the gauntlet at my feet. Now she seemed to be waiting for me to take responsibility for the fallibility of the entire medical world and the pharmaceutical industry to boot.

I ran through the scientific possibilities first. Medication side effects are certainly common, but patients usually have a specific reaction to a particular pill based on the unique properties of that medication. It stretched biological plausibility to experience reactions to nine different medications from four different categories of antihypertensives, each with entirely unrelated mechanisms of action.

Some patients are exquisitely sensitive to the slightest hiccup in their well-being and abandon pills by day two. Others are more tolerant and find that many reactions self-resolve once they allow their bodies to get used to a medication. Mrs. Ruger's symptoms could be real, or could be unrelated, or could be any mix in between. Offering these opinions to her, though, likely wouldn't get us anywhere. No doubt she'd heard all of these before, and they'd obviously not eased her dissatisfaction. The best strategy in these cases, I've found, is to remain open-minded and simply ask the patient to elaborate.

I nodded slowly as she unleashed another textbook's worth of symptoms. "Are you sure that it's the pills that are making you sick?" I then asked.

"Of course," she snapped indignantly. "As soon as I start taking them, I get sick. Sick!! When I stop, I feel better." She pursed her lips, drawing them up into a lasso of spackled pink.

I tried again. "Does every *single* pill make you sick?"

She seemed surprised that I would be surprised. Her tone was delicate but it was clear that she'd taken offense. "I have a very sensitive constitution," she replied with a sniff.

I endeavored to keep my skepticism in check. Instead, I asked her if there was any medicine that she *was* able to tolerate. Mrs. Ruger brightened immediately and said she had no trouble with the prednisone pill she took every day for her asthma.

Prednisone? *Prednisone?!* Of all the pills in her regimen, of all the pills available on the market, of all the pills in the world, prednisone carries one of the longest and harshest lists of side effects. Hardly anyone takes prednisone without experiencing side effects, many of which can be catastrophic. A steroid, prednisone causes people to feel loopy and sometimes induces frank psychosis. It upends the body's regulation of glucose and with prolonged use can push people into diabetes. It jangles the exquisitely calibrated threads of communication that link the pituitary gland, the hypothalamus, and the adrenal glands. Acute adrenal insufficiency caused by steroids has landed many a patient in the ICU. Prednisone also mutes the immune system, allowing infections to flare ferociously, sometimes dredging up dormant infections from decades past. It thins the bones, causing osteoporosis and subsequent hip and spine fractures. Along the way prednisone deposits unwanted fat in unwanted locations, leading to pregnant-looking bellies, buffalo-hump shoulders, and faces swollen to moon-shaped proportions. Almost no one escapes prednisone unscathed.

Prednisone is the one medication that doctors try desperately not to prescribe. If it's absolutely needed, then we gingerly give the lowest possible dose for the shortest possible duration. And here was Mrs. Ruger, taking it contentedly every day for years.

I had to admit there was something poetic about the irony of it all. The blood pressure pills that are dispensed so freely, and generally with so few ramifications, Mrs. Ruger could not tolerate. But the one medication that is prescribed with such reluctance and trepidation, she seemed to have no problem with. Yes, medicine is a science, but as Wendell Berry put it, "Medicine is an exact science until applied."[1] As I pondered the prednisone paradox, Mrs. Ruger's voice abruptly crumpled. "I'm sorry, doctor," she stammered. "I know I am a bad patient."

A bad patient? I was startled by the unexpected change in tone, and even more by her choice of words. But before I could even say anything Mrs. Ruger's lips began to quiver, and a tear crept out from the corner of one eye. "I'm really a terrible patient. I can't take any of the medicines you doctors give me, and I know you are angry with me."

Before I knew it, she was crying outright, saying how sorry she was that she was a bad patient, that she couldn't follow her "doctors' orders." That she was going to die from a heart attack or stroke because she couldn't take her blood pressure pills.

I leaned forward and placed one hand over Mrs. Ruger's, which were still folded around the handle of the cane. What could I say to comfort her? Telling her that it seemed odd to be able to take something as problematic as prednisone but not nine other, far more benign medications would not be constructive. And of course I absolutely agreed with her that she could indeed suffer a heart attack or stroke if she lived with a blood pressure of 200/110.

As I looked at her, eye makeup dripping beyond the frontiers of her red glasses, it dawned on me that we'd been focusing only on Mrs. Ruger's hypertension, and not on Mrs. Ruger. And that these were not at all the same thing.

Maybe we just hadn't come up with a medical regimen that agreed with her. Or maybe the blood pressure treatment was not the main issue at all. I told Mrs. Ruger that her blood pressure was a separate thing from her as a person. Just because her pressure was 200/110 and the pills made her sick didn't make her a bad person or, frankly, *any* kind of person. If we happened to find the right pills for her and made those numbers come down, she wouldn't suddenly be a "good person"; she'd still be Bernice Ruger, just with better numbers.

Mrs. Ruger sniffed and started rubbing the handle of her cane like a talisman. She wiped her nose with a tissue. "I . . . I like that," she said. And then she repeated, like a mantra, "I am not my blood pressure."

I asked if there were any stresses at home.

Mrs. Ruger was quiet for a long time. And then she started talking about how she was struggling to make ends meet. That since her Sheldon had died, she was making do with a tiny Social Security check, and that even with Medicare, her medical bills came to almost half of her monthly check. She used to live modestly well, but her life had been edging downward each year. She felt like she was trying to survive week to week, eking out an ever more circumscribed existence.

We talked for a little while longer, then agreed to focus on three distinct issues: her financial concerns, the stress she was experiencing, and, lastly, her blood pressure. For the first issue, we made an appointment for her with our social worker about her Medicare. For the second, I suggested she join her local senior center for more companionship, and then tentatively raised the issue of antidepressant treatment. She surprised me by saying she'd taken a pill for depression a few years ago and didn't have any problem with it at all. She'd actually felt good while taking it.

And for the final issue—the blood pressure—we walked through the list of all the blood pressure pills, hunting for the one that was the least problematic of all of them. We made a plan to try that one again, at the very lowest dose, taking it only every other day. I warned her not to expect perfection with it, telling her that she might need to tolerate some side effects.

I was surprised at how easily a difficult patient encounter could meliorate. It was a simple lesson that Mrs. Ruger had offered, but one that I should probably keep posted above my desk: the patient is not the same as the illness.

It was also a reminder that the pivotal issues are often lurking below the surface. To paraphrase Freud, sometimes blood pressure is indeed just blood pressure. But so often in medicine, a given symptom is just the starting point for the real issues on a patient's mind.

To probe the relationship between the starting point and the real issue, a group of researchers videotaped more than two thousand patient visits in nine cultural regions of Europe. They interviewed the patients both before and after the visits and concluded that "unexpected agendas" emerged in one out of every six to seven visits.[2] These unexpected agendas could be medical, social, or emotional, but the frequency was illuminating. In practice, this means that on a typical day for a doctor, there will be several patients for whom the meat of the visit is not easily accessed.

The researchers tried to identify the factors that made some doctors better than others at discovering the underlying agendas. Female doctors were no better than male doctors. The age and experience of doctors didn't seem to play a role. Nor did dealing with male patients versus female patients. Surprisingly, doctors who spent more time with their patients weren't any better, either.

Instead, it was the breakdown of the time that mattered. Doctors who spent a greater proportion of their time listening were the most successful. These doctors also spent a greater proportion of their time building rapport. And when they gave medical explanations, they were more patient. Nothing is rocket science here, but the outcome is crucial: if even one additional underlying agenda is sussed out on a given day, that's one less patient lost in the muck of misdiagnosis and dissatisfaction.

When I talk to medical students and interns about this sort of approach, I refer to these skills as money-in-the-bank skills. They may seem more time-consuming—initially many can be—but they are crucial investments that pay ongoing dividends in terms of effective medical care. These skills make you much more "efficient" as a doctor because you are more likely to get to the heart of the matter sooner. You end up sparing yourself and your patient endless medical circling, unnecessary testing, repetitive medical evaluations, and mutual frustration. The payoff can come within minutes and it may last for years.

Nevertheless, teasing out the underlying agenda remains challenging. Just keying into the fact that there *is* an underlying agenda is hard. The patient may not even be aware of the issue until it reveals itself. Or the hint is there but doctors gloss right over it. And even if doctors do sense that something else is going on, creating an environment that makes a patient feel comfortable enough to reveal a sensitive issue isn't always so simple.

———

Carmen Padilla, a thirty-seven-year-old woman, came to my clinic because of a scalp condition. She was casually but fashionably dressed, with well-manicured nails and carefully applied makeup, though the broad bill of a red baseball cap obscured most of her face. Thick tresses of silky black hair slid out from the sides as she shyly removed the hat. I could see reddened, crusted patches on her scalp, with rings of hair loss around them.

Ms. Padilla was the American-born child of Dominican immigrants. She worked in a bodega and was raising two children on her own. It was evident that her scalp condition was profoundly embarrassing, and she slapped the cap back on as soon as I had examined her head. I reassured her that this was a common fungal skin infection and was very easy to treat. To give her some distance from this clearly uncomfortable topic, I quickly moved onto the other parts of the medical interview: past medical history, past surgical history, and so forth.

During the course of my questioning, Ms. Padilla mentioned offhandedly that she had been having aches and pains in her left knee, her right shoulder, the back of her head, and her stomach. She said she'd had pins-and-needles sensations in these areas for the past six months.

I performed a thorough physical exam but found nothing amiss: there was no swelling in the joints, there was normal sensation in the skin, there was no sign of trauma or injury. I could find nothing to link these symptoms to any known disease. "It's probably just the routine aches and pains of life," I said. "You are perfectly healthy."

She gave a tight smile and we talked for a few minutes about general steps to maintain good health: a Pap smear, a balanced diet, exercise. I gave her a prescription for an antifungal medication to treat her scalp, and then we shook hands and said good-bye. I turned back to my paperwork as she let herself out of my office.

A minute later I heard a quiet "Doctor?"

I looked up from my writing. Ms. Padilla was standing outside the office, her hand on the doorknob, getting ready to shut the door. "Can I ask you a question?"

"Sure," I said, putting down my pen.

Ms. Padilla paused, and from under her baseball cap she seemed to focus on a spot beyond me. Her voice grew more tentative. "Do you think . . . ?"

She hesitated again, her eyes drifting, as if searching for another, perhaps safer, spot upon which to rest. "About the parts that hurt me: my knee, my shoulder, my head, my stomach . . ."

Her lower lip retreated ever so slightly under her front teeth. "Do you think it's possible . . ." She hesitated again. "Do you think it's at all important that these are the same spots where my boyfriend shot me with a dart gun?"

Bringing up new concerns toward the end of a medical visit is very common—it happens in one in five visits.[3] But the hand-on-the-doorknob phenomenon is a special case, well known to all doctors. A physician can proceed assiduously through a detailed history and physical with a patient, but it is only when the patient is halfway out the door that the important information spills out.

Why is it that the most crucial information remains hidden until after the visit has completely finished? Perhaps it is because the formality of the standard doctor-patient visit precludes revealing such personal, vulnerable details. Or maybe such details feel out of place because they aren't about spleens or triglyceride levels. Maybe only when patients are fully dressed and standing upright, physically removed from the medical setting, if only by a few feet, do they regain enough humanity and strength to reveal such things. Or maybe it's the sudden urgency, the pressing realization that a door is about to close—literally and figuratively—and this is the last possible moment to bring this secret to the fore. Whatever the reason, there is something about that moment—halfway out the door, halfway transitioned out from the odd cocoon of the medical world, halfway back into the world where your symptoms are yours and yours alone—that is galvanic. The hand on the doorknob is the last slip of connection.

There was a long pause as Ms. Padilla's dark eyes finally settled on mine. I wanted to kick myself; how could I have missed this? Why wasn't my radar alert to domestic violence? Why didn't I catch the tautness in her smile? Why hadn't I keyed into the withdrawn demeanor coupled with the seemingly random symptoms? Domestic violence is so frighteningly common that, statistically, every single day I should have at least one patient who has experienced it. Why hadn't I thought to ask?

I stood up and extended my hand to Ms. Padilla, to invite her back in from the outside, to pull her back from across the threshold. It was time for the real visit to begin.

Ms. Padilla's story is not at all unusual—not in the occurrence of the violence, nor in its invisibility in the medical setting. Data suggest that one in four women and one in seven men have experienced domestic violence at some point in their lives. The numbers are even higher when looking at the subset of people who present to the medical system—approximately 40 percent of patients who visit general family practices or emergency rooms have experienced domestic violence.[4] Up to a third of emergency-room visits by women can be attributed to domestic violence—ranging from acute injuries to complications in pregnancy to symptoms arising from the relentless stress these patients live with.[5]

There are many medical concerns that are similarly uncomfortable for a patient to bring up with a doctor. No one thrills to discuss erectile dysfunction, vaginal discharge, rectal bleeding, urinary incontinence, or loss of libido. It's rare for anyone to proudly proclaim that they feel depressed, or have an eating disorder, or don't have enough money for food, or have a spouse who is incarcerated. Besides feeling embarrassed, patients often think that these situations have nothing to do with medicine so don't qualify for the doctor-patient discussion.

A few years ago I met Gaspar Navarro, a robust seventy-four-year-old. A thick shock of white hair spilled over most of his forehead, framing skin that was leathered from a lifetime of outdoor work—farming as a teenager in Mexico, construction as an adult in the United States. Concentric rings of creases bracketed his smile. Most of his family was back home, and he lived alone in a single-room-occupancy hotel. There was an air of cheerful self-sufficiency about him, and I learned that there was a crew of Central American men at the same hotel. In warmer weather they occupied the benches out front, playing dominos and canasta. He chewed habitually on a cigar but swore to me that he never actually smoked it.

Mr. Navarro carried the usual diagnoses of men of his age—diabetes, hypertension, and elevated cholesterol—along with some prostate enlargement and back pain. And he carried the usual plastic bag of pill bottles that was depressingly bulky. At this first visit, I spilled the bottles out onto my desk, sorting them by disease. Mr. Navarro didn't remember the names of the medicines, but he did know that the white pill was for pressure and that there were two pills for diabetes. Something also for cholesterol and his prostate.

The visit took nearly an hour as I painstakingly explained each medication, matching the names on the bottles to the pill inside and the disease it was intended for. I cleaned up his medication list in the computer, purging expired or redundant meds, and then printed the list for him to take home—clear, organized, and, most important, legible.

Despite running over our scheduled time, I felt gratified that I'd brought some clarity to my patient's medical conditions. Plus I was meeting one of the patient-safety goals mandated by our hospital: accurate medication lists.

At our next visit I plucked out the bottle of lisinopril, the one new medication we'd started last time. "How does the new blood pressure pill feel?" I asked.

"Is that the one I take twice a day?" Mr. Navarro asked.

"No, it's once a day," I said, pointing to the label. "The metformin for diabetes—*that's* the one you take twice a day."

He pulled out the next bottle, unscrewed the top, and peered in. "I take these before breakfast."

I reached for the bottle and squinted at the label. "No, this is the one for your cholesterol. You have to take this one at bedtime."

Despite the hour we'd spent at our last visit, Mr. Navarro was clearly still confused about his medicines. This is not an uncommon occurrence in this age of polypharmacy. Patients with chronic illnesses routinely juggle eight to ten medications, often more, many of which change at each visit. So I pushed everything else aside and again devoted the entire visit to his medication list.

For the next few visits, I spent all of our time diligently reviewing his pills and medication list. I referred him to an eye doctor to ensure that the diabetes was not affecting his vision. I got him a pillbox to help him prepare a week's worth of medications at a time. I scheduled appointments with our nurses so they could review the medication plan with him between our visits.

In short, I did all the things that are recommended to help a patient adhere to a complicated medical regimen. It was more than a year into our relationship when Mr. Navarro finally told me the truth. I was typing up yet another beautifully manicured medication list to help keep him organized when he interrupted me.

"Doctor," he said, his voice faltering, "you don't have to keep giving me those lists." He looked down at his lap for a moment. "The truth is that I can't read. Not in English, not in Spanish. Nothing at all."

Though I knew illiteracy existed, there was still something unsettling about encountering it in real life. He couldn't read! No wonder Mr. Navarro couldn't keep his medications straight. And here I was, every visit printing up ever-neater medication lists in English and in Spanish, congratulating myself on the clarity and comprehensiveness of each one. These lists may just have well been wallpaper for his living room. Why hadn't I ever thought about whether or not he could read?

Some 15 percent of Americans possess only the most rudimentary reading skills.[6] That's about one out of every seven people! And when it comes to health literacy—understanding enough to make health decisions—more than a third of Americans lack the necessary skills.[7] This can occur in people who are fully literate in the English language, so can be easily missed. Low health literacy is strongly correlated, not surprisingly, with poor communication and poor health outcomes.[8] People with lower health literacy use fewer preventative services (mammograms, flu shots) and are hospitalized more often. They have trouble with medication labels and medication adherence and end up in emergency rooms more often. Illiteracy is even linked to higher death rates, especially among the elderly.

I recalled my travels to countries where I didn't speak the language and few spoke English. I'd felt so handicapped as I struggled to find my way. I felt impotent when I couldn't make my needs or my thought process known. To imagine that situation complicated by illness was frankly terrifying.

Watching Mr. Navarro fumble with his bottles, unsure which pills to take twice a day and which once a day, unnerved me. I envisioned mix-ups and potential overdoses. That he'd succeeded this far was a testament to his resourcefulness and perseverance. But I worried about his future, his ability to juggle multiple chronic illnesses and to navigate a complex medical world.

Like Carmen Padilla and Bernice Ruger, Gaspar Navarro had enfolded something painful deep within the linings of his heart. It took more than a year of our relationship before he could ease it open to me. How many more patients of mine are quietly suffering from things they hesitate to bring up in a medical visit? How many silent stories am I failing to hear?

When medical students are taught the basics of the medical interview, they are reminded to ask questions in an open-ended manner, to cast the net as widely as possible. They are also reminded to always ask, "What else?" It's a simple technique that most doctors routinely avoid because we worry about a deluge of additional concerns with no time to address them. But like the other strategies I mentioned earlier, this can ultimately turn out to be a time-saver. Lord knows I could have saved a full year of struggles with Mr. Navarro if I'd figured out earlier what was contributing to his difficulty with his meds.

But merely asking "What else?" isn't always enough. For patients like Carmen Padilla or Bernice Ruger, doctors have to keep their antennae sharp. For Ms. Padilla, I should have keyed in earlier that something wasn't adding up. Maybe I wouldn't have figured out right away that it was domestic violence, but I should have recognized that there was more to the picture. If she hadn't been courageous enough to hold onto that doorknob, I would have been just another doctor to have entirely missed this major trauma.

Similarly with Mrs. Ruger, I should have immediately realized that intolerance to every single medication likely signaled something else was going on. Sure, maybe she simply did have that exquisitely sensitive constitution, but I could have explored other possibilities, offered her the opportunity to talk about things other than her blood pressure.

After Mr. Navarro shared his painful secret with me, I opened up every one of the medication bottles that were lined up on my desk that day. We extracted a pill from each one and taped it onto a piece of paper. I drew a sun next to the ones that needed to be taken in the morning and a moon next to the ones for nighttime. I taped up extra tabs for the ones that needed to be taken twice a day. My artistic skills leave a lot to be desired, but I did my best to illustrate diabetes, the prostate, the back, and a blood pressure cuff. I numbered every entry and wrote matching numbers on the labels of the bottles. He left my office with a sheet of brightly colored pills, a rainbowlike guide that I hoped would offer him access to the medical benefits he surely deserved.

At the time, my daughter Ariel was starting kindergarten and just learning to read. I remember how she was struck with delirious joy each time a few random letters clicked into a word that corresponded with something she knew in real life. I watched her intently as she labored through the painstaking initial steps, knowing that each rung that she managed to surmount would have powerful ramifications in her life. It was a gift, really. A gift for her health. A gift for her longevity. A gift for engagement in the world. It was a gift that I wished I could convey to Mr. Navarro.

CHAPTER 12

The Language of Medicine

So often in medicine we speak in terms that make it sound like the patient is personally responsible for clinical outcomes. When cancer returns after treatment, for example, it is common to say that the patient *failed* chemotherapy, as though she or he were taking a standardized test and simply didn't study prodigiously enough. Patients who don't take their medications are labeled "noncompliant," even if they have a perfectly legitimate reason not to: the medication caused sexual dysfunction or they got to the pharmacy and the bill was $250 for thirty pills. When patients choose not to do a recommended treatment, doctors typically say the patient *refused* treatment, a verb choice that makes me think of a toddler storming away from a plate of broccoli, holding her breath until she turns blue.

Why must we use such harsh terminology?

The words that we doctors use cast patients in a very particular and often damning light. You could easily hear a doctor say, "Miriam Young has lymphoma. She failed chemo but is refusing radiation. She's noncompliant with her diabetes meds, so her glucose is poorly controlled." This makes it sounds like Ms. Young is a complete obstructionist, stamping her foot with a hail of invective every time her doctors offer her an eminently prudent recommendation.

The reality, however, could easily be that the chemotherapy available for her kind of lymphoma doesn't have much efficacy. So rather than Ms. Young failing the chemotherapy, the chemotherapy has really failed her.

And it could be that radiation offers only a 30 percent chance of remission but a 100 percent chance of debilitating side effects. So she's thought it through and decided it's not worth it. And the metformin for her diabetes roils her stomach. The lymphoma has already mucked with her appetite, so anything that takes away the pleasure of eating makes every day even more gray and tasteless. She's decided that enjoying a good meal is worth a blood sugar that's a bit high.

So is Ms. Young really *failing* chemotherapy, *refusing* radiation, and being *noncompliant* with her meds? We could just as easily say that Ms. Young's cancer is resistant to chemotherapy, she has declined radiation treatment because of low efficacy, and the side effects of her diabetes meds outweigh the benefits. Makes her sound like a much more reasonable person, right?

In reality, the lymphoma, the radiation, and the diabetes meds are neutral objects. They don't—and shouldn't—say anything about Ms. Young. As Bernice Ruger proved to me, the illness is not the person. Words that carry baggage—*failed, refused, noncompliant*—don't advance the ultimate goal, which is helping Ms. Young get the medical care that serves her best.

What are some other words in medicine that carry additional freight?

Most every patient who walks into a doctor's office gets a set of vital signs—blood pressure, pulse, height, and weight. Because it's hard to interpret the significance of weight without considering height, the more relevant stat is body mass index (BMI), which is weight divided by height squared. Anyone with a BMI higher than 25 is defined as overweight; anyone over 30 is obese.

More than a third of American adults clock in at over 30, so doctors are seeing plenty of obese patients in the office. But the word "obese" is very uncomfortable for many people. Even though it's a medical term with a specific definition, it still feels judgmental, and we often shy away from using it. (Things get even more awkward for the medical term "morbidly obese," which is used for those with a BMI of more than 40.) I've often wondered whether avoiding uncomfortable terms is actually helpful or harmful to patients.

Jane Ogden is a British psychologist who has examined this exact question.[1] She and her colleagues surveyed doctors from twenty-three practices in and around London and found that the word "obese" was routinely avoided. Doctors preferred to say things like "your weight may be damaging your health" or "you are overweight" or "you need to lose some weight."

The researchers also polled nearly five hundred patients with a simple scenario to contemplate: "Imagine that you are a patient who is experiencing joint pain and breathlessness. Your doctor weighs you and tells you either 'you are obese' or 'your weight may be damaging your health.'"

In general, patients said that being told, "you are obese" had a much stronger impact. They felt that the condition seemed more serious and the medical consequences graver. They did not, however, feel any worse toward their doctor for using that term. Their level of trust in the doctor, as well as their understanding of the condition, was unaltered.

The patients were weighed and divided into two groups: obese (BMI>30) and nonobese (BMI<30). Of all the issues that the researchers probed, the only thing that differed between these two groups was how they reacted emotionally to the two different phrases used by the doctor. The patients who were most upset when the doctor in the hypothetical scenario used the term "obese" were the ones who themselves were not obese. Patients who were actually obese were more upset when the doctor used the euphemism about weight damaging their health.

While vignettes may not exactly correspond to real life, the difference in response is intriguing. For the patients who are obese, it may feel patronizing for their doctor to use a euphemism. It may seem like the doctor isn't taking the condition seriously enough.

"No two people speak the same language," Ogden told me in an interview. "They have different childhoods, different cultures, different family backgrounds, different contexts." With doctors and patients there are additional realms of difference: Doctors have a specialized knowledge and vocabulary that may be entirely foreign to the patient. Patients are experiencing symptoms that the doctors are not, and each patient has an individualized and complex response to being ill.

Ogden noted that there is an increasing tendency in medicine to try to make patients happy. This is partly due to the salutary attention being paid to the humanness of the doctor-patient connection, but also due to the ever-burgeoning business side of medicine. In medical meccas like New York City and Boston, where you can hardly walk a block without tripping over a big-box medical center, patient satisfaction has become a red-hot economic issue. The medical arms race has exploded as hospitals compete aggressively for patients. (I work on the East Side of Manhattan, where the advertising budgets of medical institutions could probably fund a professional football team and build the stadium, too. Our stretch of First Avenue is affectionately—or sardonically—known as Bed Pan Alley for the sheer number of institutions in which your bodily afflictions can be tended.) It is, of course, laudable that patient satisfaction has become a high priority, but sometimes window-dressing efforts like fancy coffee in the waiting room get priority over things that might have an actual effect on health care, such as giving nurses paid time off for continuing education.

This effort to make patients happy, to keep them coming back, has permeated the doctor's office as well, and Ogden has wondered about the possible negative consequences. "You need *some* amount of anxiety in order to help people to change behavior," she said. Though too much anxiety, she noted, "can put people in denial." Doctors need to find that sweet spot that helps patients understand the gravity of the situation without overwhelming them.

Ogden conducted another study in which she examined the term "heart failure."[2] She found that doctors again avoided the medical term and overwhelmingly preferred euphemisms about hearts being weaker and fluid backing up into lungs (though one could argue that these are more explanations than euphemisms).

Patients were given a scenario in which they had symptoms of heart failure and were asked how they'd respond if the doctor told them they had "heart failure" or if the doctor said, "You have fluid on your lungs because your heart is not pumping hard enough." Hearing the term "heart failure" was more upsetting, but it also made patients rank the condition as more serious. This study didn't divide the patients up by their cardiac function, but it does point out that while medical terms carry baggage, so too do euphemisms.

In a third study, Ogden took a closer look at how doctors and patients navigate around the awkward words regarding excretory and sexual functions.[3] Once again, she found that euphemisms reign supreme, though more on the patient side than on the doctor side. Doctors comfortably talked about bowel function and penile discharge, while patients generally didn't offer up those terms (and sometimes didn't fully understand them). Ogden and her colleague designed a randomized trial in which the doctor would either use standard medical terminology during the consultation or would match the patient's language style, using whatever terms the patient offered.

For each patient, the doctor was randomly assigned to conduct the interview with matched or unmatched (standard medical) language. Based on the surveys filled out afterward, the patients were much more comfortable with the matched language. They felt a stronger rapport with the doctor and their distress was better relieved. When the doctor spoke their language, things were clearer.

The positive trend away from medical paternalism over the past few decades has extended toward language. One thing that was pointed out early on was that medical language often objectified patients, referring to them by their disease, e.g., "an epileptic" or "an asthmatic." In recognition that people are much more than their diseases, there has been a tremendous push away from that particular language structure, pressing doctors to refer to patients as "someone with epilepsy" or "someone with diabetes." Indeed, as Bernice Ruger's situation cogently reminded me, she was separate from her disease. She was a woman who happened to have hypertension, not a hypertensive.

However, I've noticed that many of my patients with diabetes in fact refer to themselves as diabetics. Ogden conducted a study on precisely that issue, investigating how patients respond to the term "a diabetic" versus "a person with diabetes."[4] Participants were given a hypothetical vignette in which a nurse had recalled them because lab tests indicated diabetes. In half the vignettes, they were told they had been "identified as a diabetic" and in the other half they were told they had been "identified as a person with diabetes." Then they answered an extensive questionnaire that probed stereotypes about diabetes as well as their understanding of diabetes and its consequences. The participants had been recruited so that half of them actually had diabetes and half did not.

The short answer of the study was that being told they were "a diabetic" versus "a person with diabetes" didn't have any effect on people's thoughts and beliefs about diabetes. For participants both with and without diabetes, the two terms seemed essentially identical.

This doesn't mean that objectifying patients is okay, or that doctors should go back to the dark ages and refer to patients as syphilitics or hysterics. (Though I could think of a few politicians who might be accurately described that way.) But it's a thought-provoking study that suggests that at least for diabetes, these terms may not make much of a difference. This might be because the term "a diabetic" in particular has integrated fairly thoroughly into the general lexicon so that it feels neutral. This may not hold for stronger terms that doctors sometimes use, such as referring to a patient with atherosclerosis throughout the body as "a vasculopath." (The first time I heard this appellation as a medical student, I envisioned a raging sociopath with clogged arteries charging down the hospital corridor, menacingly brandishing a bottle of simvastatin.)

At the other end of the spectrum is a term such as "cancer survivor," a phrase inspired from patient advocacy movements. Many patients clearly identify themselves with that phrase. While I appreciate the power behind such a statement, it has always given me pause because it goes back to identifying the person by the disease. In my charts, I write simply that a person "has a history of cancer," with clarification as to whether it has been in remission for x number of years or is considered cured.

I'm not sure if my avoidance of the term "survivor" is from the politicization of the term or from the overly self-conscious identification with the disease (that we don't hear, for example, from patients who've endured other arduous treatments such as organ transplants or neurosurgery). Or maybe it's simply that in the time and place where I grew up, to say "I am a survivor" had one and only one meaning—that one had lived through a Nazi concentration camp.

"Words are up for interpretation," Ogden told me. "I say things in different ways depending on who I'm talking to and what the situation is." Consciously or not, she speaks differently when she is talking to her university colleagues or to her teenage children or to the cable repairman, and these groups interpret her words differently.

Ogden concludes that doctors need to be flexible in their language and think about the effects of the words they use. Some types of language will be comforting, while other types will cause anxiety. Some will be neutral. Some will be political. Too much anxiety can be overwhelming but an appropriate amount can help a patient confront a serious illness more effectively.

Words can indeed be up for interpretation. This is something I learned during the floundering first steps of my medical career. When I was a first-year medical student, I earned a few extra dollars by working the 4 p.m.-to-midnight shift in our hospital's nursing office. If families wanted to hire a private duty nurse so that their loved one could have some additional attention, especially in the lonely overnight hours, they would bring their request to me and I would match them with an available nurse. It was a fairly mundane job, and most of my time was spent with my anatomy and biochemistry textbooks sprawled open on the desk.

I suspect the families did not realize just how frugal was my reservoir of medical knowledge, as they would unload their medical questions, concerns, worries, and occasional tears. I didn't even know enough to fake it, so I would do my panicky best to assist them while scrambling for an actual nurse so that there could be some actual medical knowledge in the mix beyond the seven foramina of the pterygopalatine fossa.

One evening, about 9 p.m., a nurse called to inform me that her patient had expired so she would need to be assigned to a different patient for the next day.

Expired? I had no idea what she was talking about. The image that came to mind was of the rubber air mattresses we'd used during family camping trips in the Catskill Mountains. When you opened the valve, the mattress would shake and shimmy as the air whistled out, deflating erratically until it was a flabby rumple of army-green rubber. In physiology, we learned that the lungs inspired and expired. The air mattress—like a set of lungs breathing out—expired as soon as the valve was opened. I tried to envision this poor patient, with some physiologic valve unleashed, exhaling a rush of air until he too was a flabby rumple.

But then it slowly occurred to me what the nurse probably meant, and I felt like a complete idiot. "You mean the, uh, patient, umm . . . died?" I asked, my words tentative in case I was entirely off base—a fairly regular occurrence for a medical student.

"Yes," the nurse snapped, utterly exasperated with my doltishness. "The patient expired. I need to be reassigned."

"Expired." The word rolled so oddly on my tongue. What a strange way to refer to death. My own experience with death at that time was limited to Heidi, the mushroom-colored cadaver in anatomy lab, whose pterygopalatine fossa I couldn't unearth for the life of me. I fumbled with the phone and the paperwork on the desk trying to figure out what to do for this nurse whose patient had expired.

Throughout my year in the nursing office, assorted pellets of medical jargon thumped into my consciousness, but none felt as bizarre to me as "expired." When I finally stepped out of the classrooms and laboratory into my clinical clerkships some years later, I began to hear the verb "expire" more frequently. The oddness had begun to wear off and it sort of began to sound like a normal word, though I always had a flashback to that night in the nursing office when I'd first heard it, with faint overtones of Coleman air mattresses.

During internship, I witnessed my first deaths of patients, and gradually, imperceptibly, "expired" ceased to sound strange. And, as the intern, I was responsible for writing the "expiration note" in the medical charts after a patient had died. Cartons of milk had expiration dates. Yogurts expired. Coupons expired. I guess people could too.

But I was still puzzled as to why we even had this word. I could understand why the general public might avoid the term "died," but why medical professionals? Weren't we supposed to be much more comfortable with the machinations of the human body? Didn't we pride ourselves on our technical accuracy and specificity? Didn't we say "umbilicus" instead of "belly button"? Didn't we prefer "epistaxis" over "nosebleed?" "Rhinorrhea" over "runny nose?" "Xerostomia" over "dry mouth?"

"Expired," though, is not a technical word. It's not on par with nomenclature such as pterygopalatine fossa that serves a specific purpose, however arcane. Expired is just a regular old word in the English language that we use in place of another one. A euphemism. I think we doctors employ this euphemism because we just don't like saying that a patient died. It forces us to face uncomfortable issues like grief or the limitations of our abilities. Expired is much easier because it sounds like just another medical function that you can reel off and then move on.

Popular culture holds that doctors become inured to death by seeing it so much. The existentialists, on the other hand, posit that seeing so much death has the reverse effect, making us ever more acutely aware of our own mortality. Over the years I've come to think that there is a little bit of both. Each time we see someone die we realize that it could be us, or our parents, or our children. We doctors are just as terrified of death as any other human being scurrying around this little planet. And like any other human, we use euphemism to shield us from that fear. But unlike others who get to indulge in gentler plays of language ("off with the angels" or "at a better place"), we need to institutionalize it as another piece of medical terminology—terminology that we are firmly in control of.

When students enter medical or nursing school, they are thrust into an entirely new culture, with an entirely new language to learn. It's estimated that they acquire some ten thousand words over the course of training.[5] These words are absorbed so fully that we often forget that many are not actually part of the English language. At a social gathering I once mentioned that a friend's father recently had an MI, and I was met with blank looks. I'd completely forgotten that

MI (myocardial infarction) is not the term that regular people use for heart attacks.

Another time, I was telling some friends about being on a delayed airplane when two of my kids were toddlers and one was an infant. I described how my children completely decompensated—and shortly thereafter, so did I. Again, blank looks. But this time I pressed my case. "Decompensated is a real word," I said, affronted. "It is the opposite of compensated." My friends, many with degrees in English literature and creative writing, begged to disagree. "Look it up in the dictionary," I insisted.

We did, and I was wrong. It was pure medicalese. When a weakened heart is just managing to hold it together—keeping the blood flowing in the right direction, keeping the organs at least modestly supplied with oxygen-rich blood—doctors say that the patient's heart failure is "well compensated." But a bout of pneumonia, or a week of missed meds, or a dalliance with a Chinese buffet ("dietary indiscretion" is the correct medical term here), and the patient has now *de*compensated, landing him in the hospital with fluid gurgling in the lungs, tree-trunk legs, and critical organs gasping for oxygen.

Even as I write this, my computer continually flags "decompensate" as a misspelled word. But if you've ever tried to tame two recalcitrant toddlers on an overcrowded, overheated airplane delayed on the tarmac for three hours while holding a cranky infant in your third hand, I think you will agree with me that "decompensate" is the exact right word. I plan to petition the Oxford English Dictionary for inclusion (as soon as I get those former toddlers and infant through middle school and high school!).

Given that there are some ten thousand new words that medical professionals have absorbed during their training, it's no surprise that there are lots of words that patients don't understand. Two British cardiologists polled patients in their hospital and found that many patients could not correctly define commonly used terms on the cardiology ward such as heart failure, stent, leaking heart valve, echo, and arrhythmia.[6] But their doctors were not aware. When polled, the doctors in the same hospital routinely overestimated how much their patients understood. One can see how easily there could be mix-ups when doctors and patients are literally speaking different languages.

The same, of course, holds for newbie students, who are often too embarrassed to admit ignorance of medical terminology. On my first day on the medical wards as a student, a senior resident offered me a clinical pearl. "Never give oxygen to patients with emphysema, even if they are gasping for air," she told me. "If you do, you'll end up intubating them." I nodded sagely, even though I was utterly befuddled by her advice. With a grand total of three hours of clinical experience under my belt, I had been pretty confident that giving oxygen and intubation were synonymous. When I later understood the magnitude of difference between slipping a flimsy oxygen tube under a patient's nostrils versus ramming a breathing tube down her throat and hooking up a ventilator because she has ceased to be able to breathe, I was shocked that I could have even stored those two concepts in neighboring cerebral gyri.

Then again, I also thought that cardiac arrest, heart failure, and heart attacks—ahem, *MIs*—were all one and the same. It took a lot of clinical stumbling, and some very embarrassing moments on rounds, until I got them all straight. Now, they are so far apart for me—the chaos of a code for a cardiac arrest, the swollen legs and lungs of heart failure, the urgent cardiac catheterization for an MI—that I'm flabbergasted that I'd ever viewed them as synonyms.

A good fifteen years or so after my stint in the nursing office, I was an attending physician on the medical wards. I was supervising during the month of July with a team of new doctors so fresh out of medical school that the ink was not even dry on their diplomas. There was one intern who hailed from below the Mason-Dixon Line, something of a rarity in our hospital. Her quaint mannerisms and charming Southernisms added a bit of graciousness to our brass-tacks, New-York-minute morning rounds.

One morning she came up to me, her eyes heavy, and reported that Mr. Gonzalez had "passed" during the night. My first reaction was to ask whether it was gas or stool that Mr. Gonzalez had passed, since we'd been concerned about his intestinal function. Then it dawned on me what she was saying.

"Oh, you mean he expired?" I said matter-of-factly.

She looked up at me awkwardly and narrowed her eyes. There was a long and palpable pause. Then she nodded slowly as she gradually comprehended my choice of words, which at this point were reflexive for me. I recognized in her the same uncomfortable transition I'd had those many years ago, when my everyday words for dying were replaced by the medically acceptable terms.

The experience reminded me of a story we published in the very first issue of the *Bellevue Literary Review*—the literary journal from New York University and Bellevue Hospital that I edit. It was a wonderful story by Cori Baill titled "Cousin Esther Goes to Chicago." A new intern at a Baltimore hospital is overwhelmed by all the illness around her and has trouble prioritizing her workload. She administers overwhelmingly intensive care to an elderly patient—Esther of the title—who has terminal cancer and is hardly responsive at this point. The hospital housekeeper is a local Baltimore cousin of the patient and endeavors to keep an eye on Esther's care. The housekeeper mops frequently in cousin Esther's room, watching the intern struggle to figure out what to do.

The chief resident, however, wants the intern to focus her attention on the more active patients and not squander so much time with Esther, who is nearly dead. But he's not completely heartless. "That poor woman should have already gone to Chicago," he tells the intern, trying gamely to convey his empathy as well as the local slang for expiring. The housekeeper is duly mopping the floors while this conversation transpires, thinking about cousin Esther's impending death. The story concludes with the housekeeper wondering whether in Chicago, if someone dies, they say that the person "has gone to Baltimore."

My intern's use of the term "passed" also brought to mind a favorite poem of mine, "Gaudeamus Igitur."[7] Written by John Stone, a cardiologist from Atlanta, it was delivered as a commencement address

to a class of Emory medical students who probably didn't realize just
how fortunate they were. The Latin title translates to "Therefore Let
Us Rejoice" and I've read this poem to countless students and interns
because it speaks to the emotions of moving on in medical training
and in life. It includes these lines that give a nod to the board exams
that all medical students take at the end of their schooling.

> For this is the end of examinations
> For this is the beginning of testing

I've always loved how the poet so perfectly captures the transi-
tional moment from studying to be a doctor to actually becoming a
doctor. He looks at language from two sides, in ways that remind me
of how doctors and patients often see things from different perspectives. But then he goes on to say:

> For Death will give the final examination
> and everyone will pass.

When Dr. Stone died in 2008, I thought of that line. I know he
would have been relieved that he didn't fail. Or now that his expiration date has passed, maybe he's simply gone to Chicago. Or to
Baltimore. Either way, I'm sure he knows what I mean.

CHAPTER 13

Rushing to Judgment

I had to be honest—I was uncomfortable with my new patient, a woman in her late thirties who was in my office for a general medical checkup. Maria Vincent was petite in stature but massive enough in width to meet the medical criteria for morbid obesity. Her pendulous belly hung like a third appendage between her legs and impeded her gait. A lovely-featured face was entirely swallowed up in layers of neck and jowl. Her arms could not hang straight down at her sides because of her girth.

She struggled onto the exam table, and the table shuddered under her 350 pounds. When I parted her gown at the back to listen to her lungs, waves of adipose tissue spilled over in tiered layers, muffling her breath sounds. When I palpated her abdomen, my hands were engulfed and I could not even attempt to feel her liver. Nor was I able to find her thyroid or the lymph nodes of her neck.

My job is to be nonjudgmental but the reflexive discomfort I was experiencing was impossible to deny, and I was upset at my unease. Many studies have shown that doctors display a pronounced bias against obesity—they have less respect for obese patients[1] and they develop less rapport with them.[2] The optimist in me would have hoped that medical professionals who pride themselves on caring for the ill and the vulnerable would do better than the rest of society, but alas we don't. I guess I shouldn't have been surprised, but I was dismayed. Why do doctors react that way? (Interestingly, patients have the same obesity bias toward doctors. Patients, no matter what their weight, express less trust in doctors who are obese.)[3]

No doubt one reason is that obesity—like alcoholism and drug use—is viewed as self-induced, even by doctors who are well aware of genetics and the other confounding factors involved. From the perspective of a group singularly steeped in the discipline and deprivation that got us through medical training, it's hard to jettison the idea—despite mountains of scientific evidence to the contrary—that these medical conditions could be effortlessly alleviated by just a slightly brisker sense of self-regulation.

Perhaps in obese patients we see the feared reflections of ourselves, should we lose our carefully honed discipline. My own adolescent battles with weight and body image, however modest compared with my patient's, left me with an aversion to junk food and overeating. Maybe Ms. Vincent represents my worst nightmare, what I would become if I ceased being vigilant and lost control altogether.

Maybe the pure physicality of obesity is the issue. In a society that worships svelte bodies to an unhealthy extreme, even someone like Ms. Vincent—well groomed, tidy, with an attractive face—can be perceived as slovenly just because of her weight.

These reactions are entirely irrational, of course; but emotions were never billed as rational, and doctors are as susceptible as anyone else. I don't want to be the type of doctor who prejudges her patients, and I certainly don't want to contribute to the very tangible stigma that obese people face. Yet I couldn't help my unease as I struggled to examine Ms. Vincent in my office that day.

The more I actually talked with Ms. Vincent, however, the more manageable things became. She spoke of the stress of raising children while tending to her own medical problems, many of which she recognized stemmed from her obesity. She admitted she had trouble controlling her eating and that stress only caused her to eat more. Being overweight made her depressed and that depression made her crave sweets. She related a family history of obesity, emotional abuse, and neglect. She talked forthrightly about how humiliating it was to go to the gym, and how it was nearly impossible to even find gym clothes in her size. Getting a job was hopeless: "No one ever calls back a fat person for a second interview." She couldn't reach around to her back to scratch an itch. And if one of her kids made a beeline on the street, she knew she couldn't keep up.

The more she spoke, the more my feelings moderated. Initially I'd just seen a very obese patient. By the end I saw a nuanced, exquisitely human person who suffered terribly from the obesity that overwhelmed her life. After we finished our visit, I pondered my initial response to her. Was it any different than racism, any less repellent? Even if her condition was self-induced, even partly, how could I countenance how I reacted?

Like most doctors, I like to think I treat all my patients equally, but I know that it's not true. Medicine carries a long and shameful history of ill treatment, particularly toward racial and ethnic minorities, though it has exhibited equal-opportunity bigotry toward women, gays, transgender patients, immigrants, drug addicts, uneducated patients, obese patients, patients with HIV—pretty much anyone who falls outside the rigid lines of the medical establishment. Disparities in health care have been extensively documented.[4] African Americans and other racial and ethnic minorities consistently receive less-aggressive cancer treatment, fewer cardiac catheterizations, fewer screening tests, less mental health treatment. The list is depressingly long.

Some of the disparities can be accounted for by—though not excused by—socioeconomic differences and unequal access to care. However, these two things contribute only a portion of the inequity; there are many other components in the mix. Given how essential communication is to the parlaying of medical care (in many cases it *is* the medical care), I wondered if the way doctors and patients speak to one another could explain some of the disparities in medicine.

Debra Roter and her colleagues undertook a number of studies to address this question. Using the RIAS system, they analyzed the medical visits of 61 doctors and 458 patients in the Washington, DC, metropolitan area.[5] Roughly half the patients were white and half African American. In all the encounters—as expected from other studies—doctors dominated the conversations, taking up more speaking time than the patients. (The doctors, incidentally, were about half white, a third African American, and the rest Asian.)

However, doctors were much *more* verbally dominant with African American patients than with white patients; they spoke 24 percent more than their white patients, but 43 percent more than their African American patients. The encounters with African American patients were correspondingly less patient-centered than the encounters with white patients. The overall emotional effect of the visit was also lower (less positive tone of voice and general positive emotions). You could see why African American patients often walk away from their experiences in the medical system with a worse feeling than white patients do.

Did it matter if the doctors and patients were of the same racial or ethnic group? In a separate study, the same researchers analyzed 252 doctor-patient encounters with this question in mind.[6] When doctors and patients were "race-concordant" (African American patients with African American doctors, white patients with white doctors), the visits were longer by about 10 percent. Patients rated the experience and their doctors' communication skills higher compared with patients who saw doctors of a different race. The overall emotional tone and affect were more positive.

But there was no difference in the actual communication skills. Verbal dominance was no different (doctors hogged time equally with patients of the same race or a different race). There was no difference in measures of patient-centered communication: eliciting the patients' thoughts, involving the patients in decision-making, and so on.

But patients *perceived* that things went better when they saw doctors more like them, and ultimately rated the experience higher. This may be from the comfort of familiarity. Perhaps patients—and doctors—are more relaxed in such a situation, leading to a more easygoing conversation. Or maybe it has to do with more deeply ingrained attitudes, some of which are entirely unconscious.

While there are still blatant racists out there, explicit racism is increasingly unacceptable in our society and you don't see as much of it in daily life compared with years past. However, unconscious racial bias is still an obstinate challenge and probably underlies many of the inequities we see in health care and in society at large. This is an intriguing but uncomfortable area of inquiry, as it threatens the Hippocratic ideals that medicine holds up as its paragon of professionalism.

The test that researchers use most commonly to uncover unconscious bias is called the Implicit Association Test, or the IAT.[7] The test is clever, and relatively simple—at least at first. In round one, the program asks you to rapidly classify photographs of faces as either European American or African American. The classification is done by pressing one button on the left side of a keyboard or a second button on the right. The photos are unambiguous and the task is easy. Round two has you rapidly classify words as "good" or "bad" using those same two buttons. The words are similarly unambiguous and easy to classify quickly ("joy," "love," "peace" versus "agony," "terrible," "horrible").

Now things get tough. For the next round you get a random mix of words and photos to classify—good or bad words, African American or European American photos. But there are still only two buttons. So now each button has to represent two unrelated categories together. It's tough because first your brain has to register whether you are seeing a word or a photo, and then has to decide which category it falls into (black/white or good/bad), then decide if it goes to the left or the right button. You are supposed to do these as swiftly as possible, without stopping to think.

The rub of the test is that it mixes up the associated categories. In one round, you have to press the left button for any faces that are European American or words that are bad, and the right button for faces that are African American or words that are good. In another round, it pairs them in the opposite way: the left button is for African American faces or words that are bad and the right button is for European American faces or words that are good.

The assumption is that you will do better when you have a stronger internal association between two otherwise unrelated categories. If you classify more accurately when one button associates European American with good than when the button associates African American with good, then you are felt to have a certain amount of "white preference," and vice versa.

Versions of the test have been created to test implicit bias regarding women, Muslims, obese people, Native Americans, Asians, disabled people, and skin tone. It's not a perfect measure of reality, of course, but it does offer some sense of our unconscious biases.

To elucidate if and how implicit bias might affect medical communication, researchers administered the IAT to 40 doctors and then audiotaped visits of these doctors and 269 of their patients.[8] The higher the doctors scored on the measures of implicit racial bias, the worse their communication was with African American patients. There was more verbal dominance, less patient-centeredness, and less positive affect. These patients rated their experiences with distinctly low marks.

For white patients, a higher level of implicit bias on the part of the doctor (against African Americans) was also associated with more verbal dominance by the doctor. But the white patients did not experience the visit as poorly. They actually rated their experience more positively. Thus, implicit bias was associated with poorer communication skills on the part of the doctors to all patients. But the perception of poor communication differed between white and African American patients.

Another study from the Midwest polled nearly 3,000 patients of 124 doctors who'd taken the IAT.[9] Doctors with higher levels of implicit bias again did not do well with their African American patients. These patients gave their doctors low marks when it came to patient-centered care. And white patients, as in the previous study, gave these doctors higher ratings, despite the implicit bias. Interestingly, Hispanics gave their doctors the lowest ratings of all, and, further, their low ratings were entirely unrelated to the doctors' level of implicit bias.

When doctors as a group are evaluated for implicit bias, white physicians do worse than African American physicians. Male physicians show more bias than female physicians. African American physicians, it turns out, do not show any bias on these tests; that is, they do not demonstrate an unconscious preference for (or bias against) any race.[10]

I don't think anyone is surprised that unconscious or implicit bias is prominent in medicine, even among doctors who are paragons of egalitarianism. And I don't think it's a surprise that African American patients pick up on this and come away with a more negative view of medical care.

This negative response can feed on itself and impact the experience of future medical visits.[11] A group of 350 patients about to see their doctors were interviewed about past experience with race and class bias. The medical visits were then audiotaped and the doctor-patient communication was analyzed. For African American patients who'd experienced more race and class bias in the past, the visit demonstrated more negative affect from both doctor and patient—compared with African American patients who'd experienced less bias in the past, and compared with white patients. In post-visit surveys, these patients felt that the doctors were not listening to them and were not treating them with respect.

The researchers hypothesized that past bad experiences prime patients for another bad experience by setting low expectations and giving the patient a more negative overall affect. Doctors can unconsciously pick up on and then mirror that affect, leading to a downward spiral of poor communication and connection. One potential solution is to make doctors aware of this unconscious dynamic. Perhaps by noticing the downward spiral as it's starting, doctors can make an extra effort to make their affect more positive and set the interaction on a more positive course.

Positive affect may sound like cheery window dressing but it is a critical component of communication. When expressed genuinely, it evinces a confidence in the other person. Thinking back to the "co-narrator" research of Janet Bavelas, the positive affect and confidence from one person will enhance the story told by the other person. So it's not a surprise that both white and African American patients are more likely to trust doctors who speak with positive affect.[12] For African American patients, this holds even for patients who'd experienced prior bias (who are generally less likely to trust doctors). This is not to say that positive affect makes for a better doctor, but a trusting relationship is essential before good medical care can have the chance to flourish.

In an interesting study designed to see if implicit bias can be overcome, nurses were shown videos of patients who were visibly experiencing pain and asked to decide how much pain medicine to administer.[13] When the nurses were instructed to use their best clinical judgment, they ended up giving less pain medicine to the African American patients than to the white patients. However, when the nurses were instructed to imagine how the pain was impacting the patients' lives, they ended up giving the same amount of pain medication to all patients, regardless of race. Taking another person's perspective is the building block of empathy, and this may be one of the prime factors needed to help eliminate disparities in medical care.

Clearly much systemic work needs to be done in the medical system to address inequities in care—everything from where hospitals are built and how patients get insurance to who gets into medical school and how research dollars are distributed. In terms of what individual doctors and patients can do, much of it depends on one-to-one communication. For doctors, recognizing their unconscious biases is a formidable but necessary step. Eliminating unconscious bias is not easy, but making a determined effort to see the other person as a unique individual and then taking the next step of envisioning that person's perspective can make a tangible difference. For patients—who in an ideal world shouldn't have to do *anything* to get their doctors to treat them equitably—allowing doctors to get to know them as a person offers fertile ground for empathy to develop.

Jose Santiago was a patient of mine some years ago. He'd done time at Rikers Island, though he never told me the reason for his incarceration. He possessed the craggy, almost grandfatherly look of someone who had survived—and was now officially retired from—the drug-addled 1980s. His skin was corrugated from years of injecting and his tattoos had faded to a murky bluish-gray. His raspy voice came across as exhausted but steady.

Like all new admits to Rikers, Mr. Santiago had been given a standard battery of tests for the medical ailments that run rampant behind bars. He received the unwelcome news that he was HIV positive, though luckily his T-cell count was still in the normal range. He also discovered that he had hepatitis C, plus diabetes and hypertension. He required massive doses of methadone to combat his heroin habit. What made his life most miserable, though, were the stubborn leg ulcers from his old skin-popping habit. Like many addicts of the day, when he ran out of veins, he'd simply injected drugs right into the meat of his limbs. These ulcers never seemed to heal.

When Mr. Santiago was released from prison, he made his way to our hospital's HIV clinic. He was surprisingly reliable with his complicated medical regimen and he showed up for all of his appointments. However, he didn't get the frequent lab tests to monitor the progress of all of his diseases because his veins had been obliterated by decades of drug use.

About once a year he'd allow his methadone doctor to draw blood from a ragged vein in his neck, and that was the extent of the medical evaluation that was possible. Despite the many medical assaults on his body, his immune system remained intact. His T-cell count stayed high enough to protect him from opportunistic infections (this was before viral load was easily measured, so we checked only T-cell levels).

In those days before super-strong antiviral medications turned HIV into a manageable chronic illness, it was a rare—and celebrated—circumstance to be one of the lucky "nonprogressors." I'd had only one other patient in my practice who was a nonprogressor, and it was as though a fairy godmother had surveyed the vast, dismal landscape of AIDS and selected these two patients to sprinkle with fairy dust. Such patients were beacons of hope in an otherwise bleak chapter in medicine.

With such infrequent blood draws, it was hard to follow the vagaries of Mr. Santiago's health, but he continued to have robust T-cell counts—year after year. One year the nurse practitioner who had been monitoring him in the HIV clinic made a special request. When it came time for the annual blood draw from that very last standing vein in his neck, the nurse asked the methadone doctor not just for a T-cell count but also for a new HIV test. She just had a hunch.

Lo and behold, it came back negative; Mr. Santiago did not have HIV. The initial HIV test at Rikers had been a false positive, and the diagnosis had been wrong all along. Mr. Santiago was promptly discharged from the HIV clinic and sent to the general medical clinic, where I became his doctor.

When we first met, I was astounded by the story, amazed that the misdiagnosis could have persisted for so long. I wondered why we chose to explain his vigorous T-cells by classifying him as a nonprogressor, rather than considering that his initial HIV test might have been incorrect. Was it that we put too much faith in the test's objectivity? Or was it simply that Mr. Santiago fit the HIV picture so perfectly—Rikers prisoner, drug user, hepatitis C, tattoos—that we never imagined he could be negative?

When Mr. Santiago and I began working together, his calves were filleted open from knee to ankle. These ulcers were years in the making, products of ongoing drug use in settings that were the least conducive to wound healing imaginable. At our first visit, Mr. Santiago handed me a page-long list of supplies he needed for the ulcers: sterile saline, gauze wraps, surgical tape, iodine, Silvadene cream, latex gloves, occlusive dressings—and I admit I was a little taken aback. I'd never seen an addict, even an ex-addict, so organized and responsible.

He didn't fit the picture.

Amazingly, over the ensuing years, thanks to Mr. Santiago's assiduous care, the ulcers painstakingly healed. In the end there were only thin snaking scars on his calves to mark their sites.

He didn't fit the picture.

And then one day, after nearly two decades of taking methadone at a dose high enough to knock our entire front-desk staff unconscious, he abruptly tapered himself off. Though methadone doesn't offer the high that heroin does, the body typically remains equally dependent on it and most former heroin users stay on methadone indefinitely. For many ex-addicts, methadone remains the focus of their lives ad infinitum.

But Mr. Santiago stopped the medication himself, without any fanfare. "I've had enough," he told me.

He didn't fit the picture.

When I asked him how he felt about the misdiagnosis of HIV, he simply shrugged. "It is what it is," he told me. Perhaps, given all the other things he'd suffered in his life, eight years of carrying a false diagnosis wasn't the worst thing.

Over the years, Mr. Santiago shattered myth after myth. But in reality, he didn't *do* anything; he simply was who he was. It was the medical profession that had to shatter its myths. If we'd observed the conflicting data more carefully in the beginning and if we'd examined our own biases before being so positive in our judgment, he would have been spared this brush with HIV—the stigma, the costly and unnecessary medical care, the medications and their toxic side effects.

Ultimately, Mr. Santiago bequeathed to me a profound lesson about my profession's penchant for stereotypes and snap judgments. I just wish he hadn't had to suffer all those years in the process. Once his leg ulcers had healed and he'd severed his methadone ties, he now had only the comparatively tame issues of diabetes and hypertension to contend with. (His hepatitis C had already been successfully treated by then.) Both the diabetes and the hypertension were mild and easily controlled. Without any need for specialty medical care, he eventually left Bellevue and continued with a local primary doctor near his apartment in Queens.

In one respect, Mr. Santiago was a medical success—he'd started out with a slew of grave medical issues and ended up with just two manageable ones. But in another respect, Mr. Santiago represented a failure of the medical system. In addition to the stereotypes into which we pigeonholed him—with potent consequences—there was a staggering lack of communication. I realized that I was probably just as guilty as the doctors before me who'd misdiagnosed him with HIV. Admittedly, Mr. Santiago wasn't the easiest person to communicate with. He was a laconic man of few words and seemed content to let our visits focus on his leg ulcers. I followed his lead but I'm not sure if that was a respectful mirroring of tone or a lazy acquiescence to stereotype. I recognize that I didn't make as much effort to get to know him as I usually do with my patients. Maybe my biases got the better of me; I let the florid tattoos, the prison time, and the drug history keep me at a distance. But there was a whole person inside there, someone with remarkable fortitude. I wish I'd taken the time to learn what enabled him to cultivate those traits despite the long odds. I'm sure there was much I could learn.

When I think about how doctors respond to patients who are labeled "undesirable" for whatever reason—for being homeless or drug-addicted or mentally ill or obese or malodorous—I try to make the analogy to physical discomforts that arise in the medical setting. Over the years, I've tugged off socks with lives of their own. I've changed dressings on putrid, oozing wounds. I've encountered maggots, roaches, semen, and diarrhea during physical examinations. I've felt close to vomiting many times—I'm as squeamish as the next person. I can't control my physical reactions, as I can't control some of my emotional ones. But I *can* endeavor to control what I do with them. With enough focus, I *can* tame my outer behavior.

But is that enough? Even if I hide how I feel when I am uncomfortable with a patient, my feelings still may influence how I communicate in ways that could result in poorer medical care. This is a genuine fear of mine. Will my unconscious—or conscious—biases send signals of disrespect no matter how hard I try to corral my visible reactions? Will I drive these patients away from medical care, even when these patients are often the ones who need care the most?

Modifying our external behavior and how we communicate is clearly important, but I believe we in the medical profession have a duty to work to change our inner landscapes as well. It's a tall order, I realize, but if we wish to claim the high mantle of professionalism, we need to at least be actively attempting to challenge our gut feelings. The first step is to own up: doctors and nurses need to be honest about biased feelings, however distasteful and awkward this process may be. We need to catch ourselves in the act of jumping to a conclusion, to notice that we're doing it, and then to question ourselves about the conclusions. We need to talk with our colleagues about biases in our practice to figure out where we might have blind spots. Perfection will never be achieved but that shouldn't be an excuse to resign ourselves to the status quo. The very act of paying attention, of attempting to notice our shortcomings, is how any change begins.

Another approach, to borrow a technique from behavioral psychology, is to "act as if." If a doctor can act as if an obese, or a smelly, or an irritating, or an alcoholic patient doesn't bother her, in time the uncomfortable feelings may begin to lessen. It's a bit like smiling when you feel sad—weird at first but then you grudgingly start to feel better. Pressing yourself to go against the grain is by nature an awkward action. But in time it can influence how you feel, in this case by allowing the doctor to get to know the patient better. Again, this may seem like window dressing, and if that's the only thing a doctor attempts, it will indeed amount to just that. But if it's part of a genuine effort to recalibrate how you feel and act in situations in which you might be biased, it will likely chip away at those biases. And even if the changes are only external at first, a doctor's behavior serves as a model to the students, interns, and medical staff around him. The benefits of setting the behavioral tone, even if not (yet) fully heartfelt, cannot be underestimated.

Joan Noonan was a nurse in our clinic when I started as an attending physician at Bellevue, and even she would refer to herself as an old-school nurse. She proudly wore her nursing school pin on her white coat and still treasured her nursing cap, though she joked that if she wore it to work most of the younger staff would think she was sporting a coffee filter on her head. Ms. Noonan was a nurse extraordinaire, and what stood out to me was her impeccable reverence for each and every patient. She referred to every male patient as a gentleman. She could have the most disheveled, smelly, obstreperous alcoholic ranting in her exam room and she would never utter a disparaging word. "There's a gentleman in my room who might need a little extra medical attention," she would say calmly to one of the doctors. "Do you think you might be able to pop in for a minute?" Her tone of voice was always exquisitely respectful, and it would be identical whether the patient was one of the guys who hung out near the homeless shelter on First Avenue or the president of the United

States, for whom Bellevue is the designated hospital should something untoward happen to our head of state while visiting New York City. Her attitude was genuine through and through, and the effect of her behavior on others was remarkable. You could be the most raving misanthrope on the staff and you'd find yourself inexplicably rising to her level of civility.

Respectful behavior is contagious, so even if your inner emotions haven't quite caught up yet, the actions you exhibit will inform those around you, especially if the attempt is genuine and not just a masquerade. Your subconscious will eventually be prodded along.

I was relieved to come across a more expansive population study of nearly seventy thousand patients that showed that the medical care given to overweight patients is no different than what non-overweight patients receive.[14] Despite an ingrained societal bias against obesity—one that affects physicians as well as patients—the medical profession seems to be able to deliver comparable treatment.

I'm not sure that suffices, though. Doctors may swallow their gut feelings, hold their noses, and offer adequate treatment to patients whom they deem undesirable. But that approach—even if it achieves acceptable medical outcomes—still conflicts with the foremost tenet of medical professionalism: that we treat all patients with compassion. Compassion can't be faked. It presumes genuine sentiment, within which lies respect.

When we train medical students, we talk a lot about empathy. In its most literal sense, empathy is the attempt to appreciate the emotions of another, to feel the world from their perspective. As I talked more with Maria Vincent during that first visit, I began to get a sense of what her life was like. I couldn't presume to actually *know* how she felt, but I could begin to imagine it and how I might cope with an extra two hundred pounds and the attendant stress.

When I saw her in my office recently, I felt a difference in myself. The physical exam was still somewhat uncomfortable for me (I'll be candid here) but I pushed myself to keep Ms. Vincent—the person, not the body—in the forefront of my mind. My gut emotions still pulled, but they felt more manageable.

Maybe that's what doctors should strive for: to prod our negative feelings out of the shadows, no matter how ill at ease it makes us feel. Disrespect has no place in the doctor-patient relationship. To provide good medical care, doctors must first ensure that every patient feels comfortable in their presence. If we doctors don't feel comfortable ourselves, we need to be honest about it. Only then will our biases have the chance to dissipate.

CHAPTER 14

Can It Be Taught?

"Which hand is most important in playing the cello?" my new music teacher, Peter, asked me. I had already taken lessons for a year with another teacher, so I had a reasonable handle on the basics. I took his question seriously and looked toward my right hand, which was enclosing the bow in what I hoped was an exemplary balance of tension and relaxation. I then turned toward my left hand curled around the fingerboard, fingertip pads resting on the strings in what I was fairly confident was first position.

Hmmm . . . Was the right hand driving the bow less important or more important than the left hand pressing the notes? This was probably a trick question, I finally decided. "Both," I said, sure that I had nailed him.

There was a pause to let that sink in. Then the answer: "Neither." Ha, it *was* a trick question! "It's your ear," he said. "So we'll plan to spend the next year or two working on your ear."

A *year* or two? On my *ear*?

Having grown up playing piano, I was accustomed to each note enjoying a defined, geographical place on the keyboard. On the well-worn Steinway upright that my mother bought in a junk shop for $125 the year she got married, there was no debate about where middle C lived. It was in that spot when the original ivory keys were installed in 1880. It was in that spot when the woefully abused keys were replaced after my mother's purchase in the 1960s. And it is still in that same spot some five decades later when my own kids plonk away on that long-suffering piano. It's been nearly a century and a half since it was first built by hand in the Steinway factory in Astoria, Queens, just across the East River from where I live now, and middle C has not budged a millimeter.

Not so with the cello. Strings are blank canvases; a C can be played in any of several different locations on any of the four strings. But, most perilously, there is no marker telling you where a given C is located. No frets like on a guitar, no white-key-black-key signposts like on the piano. You simply have to wrestle around on the strings till the green light snaps on in your head and your ear decrees, "Yes, that's a C." And if it's a humid July afternoon and you are wilting like a hypoglycemic geranium, or if it's December and your New York City radiator is blasting at inferno levels, well, that C may just meander to a new latitude. It's up to your ear—not your fingers—to find it.

Thus began for me an arduous but fascinating journey into the musical world of a stringed instrument. Yes, we focused on how the right hand should balance the bow and how the left hand should sink into the vibrato, but by far the most challenging work—as Peter had warned me—was on the ear. We had to teach it to listen more deeply, more critically, more skeptically, and with more sophistication than it had ever done before.

For example, it had to comprehend the distance between an F and an F-sharp. Aurally, the distance any F and its neighboring F-sharp is fixed, based on the physics of the sound waves. On a piano it's similarly fixed—the distance between a white key and a black key—and that relationship holds no matter where you are playing on the keyboard. But on the geography on the cello fingerboard, the distance between an F and an F-sharp varies tremendously. At the very the top of the cello, up by the fancy scroll, these notes lie a good centimeter apart. You have to spread your fingers generously to accommodate the yawning gap. Way at the other end, near your knees, those notes are practically on top of each other. They can be so close together at the very distant edge of the fingerboard that you need to shove one finger out of the way to make room for the next finger when you're playing a scale. The ear's job, then, is to discipline itself—and you—to a uniform sound distinction between an F and an

F-sharp, despite the fingers negotiating different physical distances along the continuum of the fingerboard.

It's now more than ten years into my cello lessons and it's still a work in progress. With each knottier piece that Peter assigns, the stakes grow higher. We've been working on the Elgar Concerto for longer than I've been working on this book, and he'll still nail me for flubbing the F-sharp. At the one-decade mark I'm just now getting through the second of Bach's six suites, and each movement throws an ever more fastidious wrench into my tenuous musical reserve. (And at the rate I'm progressing on the Bach, I will have burned through my entire Medicare benefits before I reach the sixth suite.) "You can't ever let it up off the mat," Peter tells me, as we slog through page after page of Bach's labyrinthine harmonic maneuvers. Tuning one's ear to listen explicitly in music, it turns out, is a never-ending process.

Twenty-five years into my medical practice, I have to conclude the same thing: tuning one's ear to listen explicitly in medicine is a never-ending process. The late John Stone—cardiologist, poet, and Southern gentleman nonpareil, whom I mentioned two chapters ago—connected these two types of listening in my favorite poem, "Gaudeamus Igitur." (It's a magisterial four-page poem, so there's ample enough wisdom to sneak in at least three quotes in every one of my books.)

> For you can be trained to listen only for the oboe
> out of the whole orchestra
>
> For you may need to strain to hear the voice of the patient
> in the thin reed of his crying.

Listening to a patient might seem like the easiest of the many medical skills that a doctor needs to master, but in fact it is one of the hardest, especially if you want to do it well. This is the conclusion that many medical schools are finally reaching, after a century of assuming that two ears affixed to a skull was sufficient preparation.

When I was a medical student, there wasn't any explicit listening training—we were simply tossed into the clinical waters. I wouldn't necessarily advocate that now, though there's certainly something to be said for jumping right in. As a beginning medical student with not a single clinical skill to offer, listening is all you have so listening is all you do. One of my first clinical encounters was at NYU's cranio-facial clinic, where young children with severe birth abnormalities undergo dozens of intricate reconstructive surgeries. I remember just listening and listening as parents recounted their harrowing journeys (and also listening to the surgeons, who displayed a sensitivity and perceptiveness I've never seen surpassed). A month later I was in a locked psychiatric ward at Bellevue as a young man with a personality disorder and active delusions delivered a theater-worthy monologue that kept me spellbound. I just listened and listened. Not long after that I was on the trauma service, listening to the story of a teenager who'd fallen out of a motorboat on a summer outing and lost both legs to the motor.

These were riveting experiences in listening, ones that I remember all these years later. But no one ever sat down with us and talked to us about the skills of listening, especially in situations where patients might be reticent to speak or key issues could be hidden beneath the surface.

Donald Boudreau is a physician at McGill University, my undergraduate alma mater, who pioneered a course specifically to help medical students develop more astute listening habits, to listen beyond the meaning of the actual words spoken.[1] Boudreau calls this "attentive listening." The first thing the faculty would do is have students listen to a short excerpt of a Scarlatti piano sonata, but they would hear three versions by three different pianists. The students were asked to close their eyes while listening and hear how three people could play the identical notes, yet sound so vastly different. After they opened their eyes, they listened to the music again but also watched a "sound graphic" that offered a stark visual representation of the sound waves and saw how different they appeared in the three versions.

Later in the course they listened to (and watched the sound graphic of) a woman with depression. Before treatment, the patient spoke slowly and in a monotone. There were long pauses between phrases and words. The volume and pitch hardly varied. After treatment, the patient's voice was animated. The pauses evaporated, and volume and pitch had normalized. Visually, the sound graphic was far more lively. Now there's nothing revolutionary here—doctors and nurses well know how different a patient can sound after depression has been treated. But for the students, this was a way to focus them very attentively on the details of a patient's speech.

Another exercise had the students pay attention to specific word choices that patients make. A patient with leukemia revealed interesting details. When the patient spoke of the healthy side of herself, she used a first-person pronoun: "I was healthy for forty-four years before this happened." But when she spoke of the illness, she often switched to third person: "People with leukemia always feel tired." In the course of a normal doctor-patient conversation, this shift likely wouldn't even be noticed. But having it specifically pointed out helps students see the distancing that patients often employ in coping with disease.

Medical schools all over are developing formal curricula in which the elements of listening and communicating are discussed. Students get to practice with one another, with standardized patients (actors), and then with real patients. Faculty give direct feedback, even on small things: did they make eye contact, did they allow patients to talk without interrupting, did they introduce themselves, did they acknowledge emotions that arose during the encounter, did they solicit the patient's opinions, did they adjust their language to match the patient's, did they check for understanding, and so on.

These are all skills that the most successful doctors and nurses have picked up over time. But there are a lot of years of bumbling that could be avoided by explicitly teaching these skills at the outset. Even just the act of focusing on and talking about these skills is salutary. It sends the message that good communication is the foundation of good medicine, not just an added pleasantry. And as the cranio-facial surgeons taught me by example when I was a beginning medical student, these skills are equally important for procedure-based doctors.

But are all these training courses effective?

A group of British researchers developed an intensive three-day training course for oncologists,[2] based on a model created by Mack Lipkin, one of my colleagues from NYU. The doctors practiced extensively with actors who simulated patients, then received wide-ranging feedback from both the actors and an experienced facilitator. They also spent time critically reviewing videos of themselves in action.

Compared with doctors who did not undergo the training, these participants demonstrated significantly more effective communication skills. Their questions to patients were less leading and more open-ended. They refrained from interrupting and were better at summarizing information for the patients. They were more astute at following the patients' leads in conversation. Probably the most impressive outcome of this training was that these doctors continued to exhibit these better communication skills, even a full year later.

One thing about communication training, as the example above demonstrates, is that it is labor intensive and expensive. Having standardized patients work one-on-one with medical students (plus a faculty evaluator) is tough to pull off when you have 150 or more students and need them to get experience with a variety of clinical scenarios. There's been a lot of interest in web-based versions of this in which trainees can watch a doctor-patient interaction, usually with a faculty member pointing out key elements of communication and how they are done well or poorly. In one study of fourth-year medical students, viewing web-based modules was associated with higher scores in their clinical skills exams (which involved interviewing standardized patients).[3]

Debra Roter and her colleagues created a similar web-based program directed at both doctors and patients.[4] They developed ten-second clips of actors demonstrating specific communication skills. For patients, the skills included things such as asking for clarification, prioritizing concerns, and setting goals for the visit. For doctors, the skills were things such as asking open-ended questions, paraphrasing what the patient had said, and asking about challenges when it comes to adherence. Both doctors and patients benefited from the training, and both reported using more of the taught skills. Patients were more satisfied with their doctor visits after both did the training. The one skill area that did not improve, interestingly, was the same for both doctors and patients: time management skills. Maybe it's time to admit we just need longer visits!

Research continues to bear out that communication can be broken down into discrete skills that can be taught and retained,[5] that one needn't be born a Nelson Mandela or Winston Churchill to do a decent job communicating. Just as doctors can be taught how to suture, how to run a code, how to hear a heart murmur, and how to brake a gurney without severing their toes, they can also be taught how to communicate better.

One area that is rightfully getting attention is teaching how to break bad news. Grave illness comes with the territory in medicine, so giving bad news is a regular event for most doctors. Not so for patients. "To the typical physician," observed Anatole Broyard in his book *Intoxicated by My Illness*, "my illness is a routine incident in his rounds, while for me it's the crisis of my life."[6] Then he noted drily, "I would feel better if I had a doctor who at least perceived this incongruity."

Bad news is usually a singular event for a patient, an ordeal of pain and shock. Being saddled with a medical event that entails bad news is horrible enough; having someone botch the delivery of that news is simply tragic.

No doctor enjoys conveying bad news and many obfuscate or sugarcoat—or avoid the situation altogether—because of their own discomfort. Whether it's their existential discomfort about mortality or just a lack of confidence in their communication skills, these conversations are often less than ideal.

Even when doctors are trying to do the right thing, they fear upsetting the patient or taking away hope or simply getting into deeper emotional waters than they are able to navigate. Often, doctors lean heavily on statistics—prognoses, five-year-survival rates, chemotherapy response rates—but this attempt to be informative can backfire.

Oncology training programs have taken up the mantle of teaching communication skills for delivering bad news, as oncologists do more of this than most physicians. A number of intensive courses have sprung up, similar to the communication workshop mentioned earlier, but it's very hard for a doctor to take a day off or a weekend away to do a training program. This is especially the case for oncology fellowships, which tend to be small and thus can't spare doctors for these training programs. The faculty at MD Anderson Cancer Center in Texas decided to create a training program on difficult conversations for their first-year fellows, with one-hour sessions on a monthly basis.[7] The one-hour sessions used case discussions, reflective writing about the fellows' own experiences, and role-playing, which not only gave the doctors practice in delivering bad news, but also allowed the doctors to take on the patients' roles and get a sense of how it feels to be on the receiving end.

Like the other training programs, this focused on specific skills of communication: attentive listening, soliciting the patient's viewpoint, expressing empathy, and avoiding false reassurance. The situations were real-life scenarios such as telling a patient about cancer, discussing end-of-life issues, transitioning to palliative care, meeting with family members, handling emotional breakdowns. Though they had only one hour per month, the doctors were able to use more of these communication skills in their subsequent clinical practice.

No matter how much training and experience doctors and nurses have, though, breaking bad news never gets easy. One time, I was taking my medical team to see a new patient in the hospital. We hadn't met the patient yet, but medically it was a straightforward admission—a fifty-year-old man getting his second round of chemotherapy for colon cancer. Unlike patients admitted from the emergency room with heart attacks or GI bleeds, this type of elective admission was relatively pro forma. The oncologists were the ones who ran the show—writing the chemotherapy orders, deciding which tests were needed, determining when the patient was ready for discharge. But these patients were nevertheless assigned a medical team to keep an eye on things. It was the clinical equivalent of babysitting—being around in case anything happened, but otherwise just being a social presence.

We stood in the hall just outside the patient's room as the intern gave a brief presentation of the case. Albert Mason was an otherwise healthy African American fifty-year-old who'd never seen a doctor in his adult life until three months earlier, when he'd noticed some blood in his stool. A colonoscopy and CT scan revealed an invasive colon cancer that had already spread to the liver and lungs—a rotten diagnosis. Although cancer treatments have improved markedly over the years, metastatic cancer is still metastatic cancer. Once the disease has infiltrated other organs it is nearly impossible to cure. Chemotherapy can shrink the tumors, improve symptoms, and even allow patients to live longer, but cancer cells are ingenious in their defenses and nearly always roar back to eventually kill the patient. For someone like Mr. Mason, with infiltration of the liver and lungs, the chance that he'd be alive a year from now was low.

The medical team hung back in the hallway before entering the patient's room. The bleak outlook, as well as our team's backseat role in Mr. Mason's care, compounded to spread a sense of resignation to everyone.

"Nothing much for us to do," the intern said grimly, and I knew that she meant it both in the long-term sense and in the practical matter of our day-to-day work. I understood her unease, but as the attending physician, I couldn't second her opinion. "There's *always* something for us to do," I told the team gamely, though inwardly I wondered if my pedagogical imperative was unduly influencing my optimism.

We trooped in and Mr. Mason eyed us as we gathered in the standard semicircle around his bed. "If I'd known we were having a party, I'd have gotten some snacks," he said with a lopsided grin, slim and young-looking in his Yankees cap. Nobody said anything.

"All I got is Ensure, if anyone's drinking," he said encouragingly. My team smiled nervously.

I asked Mr. Mason if he had any questions, if there was anything the oncologists hadn't fully explained. "Nope," he said, as he gestured to the IV pump at his side. "*I'm* the cancer expert now—ask me anything!" He took a swig of his Ensure. "And the chocolate ain't bad," he said, winking at the team.

The intern was right; there really wasn't anything for us to do. The chemotherapy was already in progress, the orders had all been written, the medical plan was fully in place. With nothing technical to talk to Mr. Mason about, I asked him how he was feeling today. "Great," he replied, rolling his shoulders like a boxer. "That first chemo got rid of everything—the pains in my stomach, the blood in the toilet." He plopped his can of Ensure on the bedside table and it landed with a resonant thunk. "I'm totally back to normal."

It was a stupendous clinical success that a single round of chemotherapy had resolved his symptoms, but something in the conviction of his voice didn't sit right with me. I changed the subject and asked what sort of work he did.

"I just finished my first season as a park ranger in Brooklyn. It's like a job sent down from heaven—being in the countryside while living in the city!" He cracked his knuckles. "First season is always probation, but if they like me, they'll hire me back next season."

Next season? The team around me shuffled awkwardly. How could he be talking about next season? Didn't he know?

Carefully, I asked him what he understood of his diagnosis.

"Well," he said, shoving the baseball cap farther back on his head. "I know that it's traveled to the liver and my lungs—they told me that. I know that it's serious, but it's not the fatal type."

Not the fatal type? I could feel the weight of his statement ricochet like a ball bearing through each member of the team. As delicately as I could, I asked if he knew what it meant to have cancer in other parts of his body.

"Means I got to do chemo every month," he said, patting the IV pump like an affectionate sidekick.

I asked him if the oncologists had explained what the chemo-therapy could achieve.

Mr. Mason rubbed a nonexistent mustache with two fingers. "I ain't never really thought about that," he said slowly. "I guess it's supposed to make me better."

The heaviness of the air was now unbearable. It was clear that Mr. Mason did not really know his prognosis. Whether this was from inadequate explanations on the oncologists' part or because he hadn't been able to comprehend what he had been told was a moot point. Here we were, a set of doctors standing before a patient with a misunderstanding of grave proportions stretched between us. I wasn't Mr. Mason's primary doctor. I wasn't his oncologist. Our team was supposed to be the backseat babysitters, but here we were. There was no backing out.

I slowed my pace of speaking to match his and explained that the chemotherapy could shrink the tumors and make him more com-fortable. But it would not—unfortunately—be able to take the cancer away completely. Once the cancer had spread to the liver and lungs, it could not be cured.

"I knew that," he said quickly, almost defensively. "They told me that."

Then he abruptly swung his legs over the side of the bed so that he was sitting up straight in front of me, the crisp whites of his eyes just inches from mine. "So, Doc," he said, letting the back of his left hand fall into the palm of his right with an audible slap, and then proceeded to deposit the million-dollar question right at my feet. "How much time I got?"

The din of the hospital suddenly dissipated, leaving a wincing silence in the room. No, there was no backing away on this one. Mr. Mason didn't sound angry or resentful, or even sad. With his di-rect, even tone and that one simple question, Mr. Mason was press-ing the medical profession up against the wall, his fingers firmly on its neck.

I closed my eyes for a moment—a reflex that sometimes happens when I need to gather my courage. There are few situations more horrible than having to tell another human being that he or she is going to die. And it doesn't get any easier with experience.

I started to tell him that the studies only give us averages, that every person is different, that it's impossible to give an exact number, that there's no crystal ball. But five medical trainees stood behind me. If I evaded the question or relied on euphemisms, I would fail them. More important, I would fail our patient. If there was ever a no-bullshit moment, this was it.

I steadied my voice. "According to the books," I said, "for people with colon cancer at your stage—stage IV—the average life expectancy..." I stopped. Even after having told this to countless patients, the words still caught in my throat. I had to force them forward. "The average is about six to twelve months."

There. I'd gotten it out. And now the numbers lay there in the open—harsh and unforgiving.

I quickly added that this was an average, that some people live longer but some shorter, that it was difficult to predict for an individual person—but these hedges sounded pathetic, even to my own ears.

Mr. Mason's left eyebrow inched up his forehead, corrugating the skin directly above. "So you're saying, Doc, that if I've ever wanted to get to Vegas—I should do it now?" His voice wasn't accusing, or even disappointed. It just sounded thoughtful.

I told him I wished I could give him better news.

"I'm a lousy gambler," he said. "But maybe I'll do better now, knowing there's nothing to lose." A pensive stillness suffused the room, and I couldn't deny the temptation to wrap up quickly and pull my team away from this awkwardness. But I knew we had to stand strong in this moment of vulnerability, fear, and hard-edged reality. We owed it to Mr. Mason. And if we had any shred of self-respect, we owed it to ourselves and to the medical profession.

Finally, collective breaths were exhaled, and as if by unspoken agreement the moment of silence drew to a close. In quieter voices, we discussed the future—when Mr. Mason might start to feel ill, what he should say to his employer, what some options were regarding health care proxy and advance directives. We talked until we'd answered as many questions as he wanted to ask. We agreed to continue the conversation the next day, after he'd had more time to think. He shook my hand firmly, then lay back on his bed, pulling the bill of his Yankees cap low over his eyes.

We filed silently out of the room. When we reassembled in the hallway, the intern slumped against the wall, visibly drained. She shook her head slowly but couldn't seem to put her feelings into words. The team awkwardly shifted papers and stethoscopes. We'd all known Mr. Mason's prognosis before we entered the room. But now that it had been put into words—given life, as it were—it was a palpable, disquieting presence among us. We had directly acknowledged death and its inevitability. Sure, death is inevitable for everyone, but it's different when there's imminence. The rest of us were free to continue corralling our existential denial, convincing ourselves that our deaths were far off in the serenely incalculable future. But not so Mr. Mason.

As with all education in the medical world, patients are the best teachers. Mr. Mason reminded us that communication is much more than just one party uttering words that fall upon the ears of a second party. The oncologists may have laid out all the facts for Mr. Mason, but he didn't or couldn't fully hear them. It's also a reminder that words are not created equal. The words of a serious diagnosis or a grave prognosis carry an emotional weight that makes them especially challenging to comprehend. This underscores the need for specific training for medical caregivers in this realm of "difficult conversations." Luckily, there is accumulating evidence that doctors can get better at this with training.

But no matter how much we prepare, these conversations never will be—and never should be—easy. These are momentous, harrowing occasions. Such conversations are among the hardest things that doctors are ever called upon to do. In some ways they define the profession: accompanying patients in these most painful transitions is what medicine, in its truest form, is all about.

CHAPTER 15

A Fragile Truce Shatters

It was a drizzly August day when I met Morgan Amanda Fritzlen in the lobby of the Loews Regency Hotel on Park Avenue. I had been corresponding with Morgan Amanda for three years at this point but we'd never met in person. We'd spoken on the phone countless times, each conversation lasting hours. Her equally gregarious and detailed e-mails usually ended with a self-deprecating apology for sending an anthology instead of a letter. I felt I knew her reasonably well, as epistolary partners go, by this time. Still, the person who greeted me somehow looked entirely different than the mental image I'd created.

Part of it may have stemmed from the fact that I'd bicycled through Midtown traffic during rush hour, ending up hot, sticky, and ultimately drenched in rain. I looked so scraggly by the time I arrived, soggy helmet in hand, that the hotel doorman gave me a skeptical once-over before reluctantly opening the door. Morgan Amanda, on the other hand, was immaculately dressed in a sweetly prim flowered dress of pale pink with a white crocheted sweater and matching purse. She looked like she was ready for a mint julep after church rather than a bone marrow transplant evaluation at Memorial Sloan Kettering.

Delicately featured, with nearly translucent porcelain skin, Morgan Amanda seemed the epitome of quiet, well-mannered Southern graciousness. Though she hadn't danced ballet since childhood, she retained the willowy grace of a ballerina—slender neck, lithe torso, and delicate, sinewy movements of her limbs. From her extensive medical history and concomitant battles with the medical system, I must have expected someone more pugnacious and bruised. But she exuded a genteel reserve, an unpretentious sweetness that was both understated and instantly likable. (Though she did e-mail me the next day to inform me that what might have appeared demure was actually a severe underdosing of her daily caffeine and that her downing of a Diet Coke when we were together was strictly for neuro-stimulatory purposes.)

We discussed the latest in her medical saga, as well as her current foray into the African American literary canon: *The Bluest Eye*, *Sula*, *I Know Why the Caged Bird Sings*. Morgan Amanda was still living in Atlanta but she had been traveling extensively to the Washington, DC, area for medical care at the National Institutes of Health and at Johns Hopkins medical center. At this point, the working diagnosis was Neuro-Behçet's disease (pronounced *be-SHET's*), an autoimmune disease in which the body's antibodies attack its own blood vessels. This was on top of Ehlers-Danlos syndrome, the connective tissue disease that had also been diagnosed, which weakened the collagen throughout her body. Her clinical condition relapsed frequently and she was spending nearly as much time in hospitals and doctors' offices as she was in school.

Morgan Amanda was receiving ongoing plasmapheresis to keep down the level of antibodies, but the procedure—meant to be temporizing but which in her case was ongoing—was fraught with infections and blood clots. The autoantibodies from the Neuro-Behçet's, in addition to causing strokes and swollen joints, were decimating her red blood cells. Her bone marrow was unable to regenerate sufficient red cells for survival, so she had become dependent upon regular blood transfusions.

Both the transfusions and the plasmapheresis required inserting catheters in her veins, which had become so scarred from overuse that they were essentially unusable. The doctors had to dig deeper and more aggressively in order to implant the necessary catheters. In one half-year period she was hospitalized four times for massive infections from all the procedures. One of these episodes was complicated by acute kidney failure from the toxicity of the big-gun antibiotics. Nevertheless, she wrote to me in an e-mail at the time, "I am still counting the abundant blessings in my life. I consider myself a realist, but I must have a ridiculous sense of optimism because I continue to pursue the medical care that will allow me to live and to live as fully as I can. Not everyone would choose what I have chosen, but that is the beauty of free will. For that and for everything and everyone else in my life, I am exceedingly grateful."

Morgan Amanda was still convinced that a complete ablation of her bone marrow (with a subsequent bone marrow transplant) was the only thing that held out hope for her unremitting autoimmune dysfunction. She was pursuing evaluations in Seattle and New York, as well as in DC—anywhere that would consider her.

After Juliet had helped Morgan Amanda obtain medical evaluations at the National Institutes of Health, they worked together for another few months. But these months were strained. Morgan Amanda was convinced that Neuro-Behçet's explained everything, but Juliet was still skeptical. Morgan Amanda's list of medications was multiplying, and she was requiring ever higher doses of pain medications to treat her joint pain. She insisted on continuing the plasmapheresis as well as the immunosuppressive infusions, and was talking about possibly getting intrathecal treatments—medications delivered directly into the spinal canal.

"She wanted to pursue extremely high-dose, high-risk treatments," Juliet said, and this was not sitting well with her. The treatments carried grave side effects and Juliet could not be sure which of her patient's symptoms were from the native disease and which were caused by the treatments.

"I have to believe things will work out as they should," Morgan Amanda wrote to me after our meeting that August, "and I look forward to hearing from the Sloan Kettering team in early September and meeting with the Seattle team in mid-September. I will conclude this paragraph with the best news I received in New York: I have up to 28 potential matches in the bone marrow registry!! What an enormous privilege."

Morgan Amanda continued to push for the bone marrow transplant and Juliet was increasingly concerned about the toxic side
effects of the treatments. At their monthly medical visits, Juliet
wanted to focus on polypharmacy, drug interactions, and damaging
side effects. Morgan Amanda, however, wanted to spend the visits
discussing the research papers on Neuro-Behçet's and bone marrow
transplants that she came armed with. The incongruity of their re-
spective agendas became increasingly difficult to navigate.

"This diagnosis of Neuro-Behçet's has completely changed my
understanding of my health issues over the years," Morgan Amanda
wrote to me during the time I was writing the initial chapters of this
book. "To be frank, it has changed my entire life—for the better, I
believe. Knowledge is power, and the devil you know is better than
the devil you don't." Then she added, with a winking emoji, "Clichés
are cliché for a reason, right? Anyway, I wanted to share that with
you, as I feel it changes my story. Hindsight is always 20/20—and
there I go again with the clichés!"

In my conversations with Juliet, she struck me as the type of
doctor who goes the extra mile to be empathetic with her patients,
and I wasn't surprised to learn that many doctors in her community refer to her the patients who have unique needs. Juliet thinks
deeply about her patients and is passionate about medicine. Her
patients have her personal phone number and know they can call
her any time.

"While I usually am very collaborative in my approach," Juliet
wrote to me, "Morgan Amanda wanted to try therapies that were
unproven for diagnoses that were not definitive, and she wanted me
to be her partner in writing orders for these treatments."

The final breakup was initiated by Morgan Amanda. At their most
recent visit, Juliet had proposed tapering off some of the medications.
Because the medications carried such wide-ranging side effects, Juliet thought it critical to figure out where the symptoms would settle
without the assortment of meds causing their own symptoms.

When Morgan Amanda arrived at what would be their last visit,
she announced that she had made the decision to leave. She needed
a doctor who was more on the same page with her. "It's a battle for

me to be under your care," Morgan Amanda said, and Juliet had to agree. It was a battle for both of them. Nevertheless, parting was very emotional—after all, they'd been through so much together. "You are a person I could be friends with," Morgan Amanda said to her doctor, with tears spilling down her cheeks. "But this isn't the doctor-patient relationship I want."

"When she left my practice," Juliet told me, "it was a painful separation for me. I had invested an extraordinary amount of energy in her care. At the same time, I recognized that she had made the correct decision." The two women did stay in touch, at least online. Things were cordial, and they connected over interesting articles and books. For medical privacy reasons, Juliet did not probe into the on-going care with her new doctors, though Morgan Amanda did update her periodically.

"One lesson learned," Juliet wrote to me later, "is that perhaps I should have recommended that she see another physician sooner, though I did not know who to point her toward. So, why did I stay? On a personal level, Morgan Amanda was an extremely compelling person—interesting, witty, beautiful, and articulate. I bonded with her over her interest in books and her sense of humor. She made a tremendous impact because of her exceptional qualities. She was also a wonderful friend and advocate for many people in the Ehlers-Danlos community. I very much wanted to help Morgan Amanda, but in the end I was terrified that she could die as a result of her treatment, and I did not want to be the person responsible for writing those treatment orders."

I understood the terrible quandary Juliet faced. As a physician, you want to do the right thing for your patient. When your patient requests something you are sure is harmful, it is agonizing—do you do what the patient wants or what you think is right? From day one in medical school, we are inculcated with the idea "First, do no harm." This is the very backbone of medicine. However, I also appreciated Morgan Amanda's desperation. And so did Juliet. "From Morgan Amanda's standpoint," Juliet observed, "her quality of life was very poor and she was willing to take huge risks in an attempt to improve it. Perhaps I never could fully understand this perspective."

As a writer, I had a unique opportunity to get to know these two extraordinary women. I was moved by their honesty and generosity. Hearing their two sides of the same events illustrated how complicated any relationship can be, but especially so when the unpredictability and vulnerability of illness are mixed in. I felt privileged to listen in on the very hard work of being a patient and the tremendous challenges of being a physician. But it was also uncomfortable because real life was playing out. This was not fiction, or even a thirdhand war story. A gap in communication with Morgan Amanda usually meant hospitalizations and medical setbacks. An e-mail would then arrive with a comprehensive, single-spaced summary at a level of detail on par with a research journal. Though the update would inevitably end with a comment such as "Well, I've done it again—written a novel of an e-mail when I intended a brief reply!"

After my meeting with Morgan Amanda in New York, I threw myself into the meat of writing this book. It began with the story of Juliet and Morgan Amanda, and I had actually written their chapters first, so I put that aside while I dug into the research and stories for the other chapters. It was a full year before I finally got the other chapters caught up and was ready to pull the whole book together. My editor suggested I interview Juliet and Morgan Amanda again, now that some time had passed since their split, to see how they might reflect back on lessons learned.

I e-mailed them both but didn't hear back from either. The silence puzzled me, as both were ardent epistolarians and natural writers. Finally I received a reply from Juliet. She apologized for the delay and said she'd needed some time to compose her thoughts. She'd attached a letter for me, which I opened with some amount of trepidation. It was two pages—single-spaced.

"Tragically," Juliet wrote, "I learned that Morgan Amanda died last month. Her mother contacted me to let me know. She had developed gastrointestinal bleeding and a colectomy was recommended but she declined, after having been through so much medical care and treatment."

It was like a soundless explosion fracturing off the page and I shivered as the reality of her words sunk in. How could . . . ? How did . . . ? It just didn't seem possible. I mean I knew, intellectually, that Morgan Amanda had a severe illness and that she was receiving treatments with frightening risk profiles. Yet her voice was so singularly imbued with optimism and confidence that it was hard to imagine that anything could get the best of Morgan Amanda Fritzlen.

I read the letter again and again, sadness spilling over in great pressing waves. In the everyday humdrum of the ordinary medical world we can sometimes lull ourselves into thinking that we have this beast licked, or that at least we've defanged the worst of it. But illness retains its ruthless talents. It drives me to fury to see it pillage. *We can best you*, I want to spit back, buttressed by the armada of medical research at our flanks. But more than the anger, more than the humbling, there's just sorrow. Lonely, unanswerable sorrow. How can a life that was so vital, so vibrant, be gone?

After Morgan Amanda left Juliet's care, she experienced a few months of stability. It was during that window that she and I had met in Manhattan. But after that, the illness flared with a vengeance. The autoantibodies of the Neuro-Behçet's attacked her intestines, the walls of which were already compromised by weakened collagen from the Ehlers-Danlos.

The antibodies corroded the blood vessels lining the gut, causing these to bleed internally. The situation was complicated by the fact that Morgan Amanda was also on anticoagulants (blood thinners) because of her repeated blood clots. The combination of anticoagulants and eroding blood vessels is treacherous. Stopping the anticoagulants risked a life-threatening blood clot. Continuing the anticoagulants risked all-out hemorrhage.

"By the time I got her to the ER," her mother told me about her first episode of bleeding, "her hemoglobin was down to 3." Morgan Amanda had lost about three-quarters of her blood supply. The ER doctor at the time had said, "I can't believe she's not dead."

Morgan Amanda underwent emergency surgery but the bleeding colon could barely be repaired because the tissue was so fragile.

She spent three rocky weeks in the ICU and scarcely managed to squeak by.

The months that followed could only be described as a relentless pounding by the illness. The intestinal bleeding repeated three more times. The extensive blood loss caused dizziness, and several times Morgan Amanda fell. The compression fracture of her spine from the most serious fall chipped away at her exquisite dancer's carriage. Pain became an ever-more tormenting facet of her life.

The Neuro-Behçet's eroded her vision. It was January when Morgan Amanda realized she couldn't see the street signs. It became clear that it was not safe for her to drive, and she had to give up her source of independent travel. Her vision steadily deteriorated until she could no longer watch TV and had to struggle to see the numbers on her cell phone to call her friends. For a bibliophile, losing the ability to read a book is perhaps the cruelest punishment imaginable.

Each time she ended up in the emergency room with intestinal bleeding, the surgeon told her she needed to have the colon removed, that piecemeal repair of the friable tissue didn't even rise to the level of a Band-Aid repair. But the idea of a colostomy bag, on top of everything else, was just too much to contemplate.

On the fourth bleed, the surgeon was adamant: removal of the colon was the only option to prevent complete exsanguination. But it was not a treatment to be taken lightly; in her weakened state, the surgery would be exceedingly risky. But *not* operating was also risky. By this point, Morgan Amanda was receiving plasmapheresis three times per week, in addition to infusions of cyclophosphamide. She had to administer bags of IV saline at home to keep herself appropriately hydrated. Because her blood count was so low (even before the episodes of bleeding), she needed ongoing blood transfusions. She was taking close to forty medications and was constantly traveling back and forth to doctors' appointments. The medical maintenance was already overwhelming. Contemplating a colostomy was just too much.

"How will I ever take care of it?" Morgan Amanda asked. There were days when she couldn't even wear shoes because the skin on her swollen feet was breaking down. An inadvertent jiggle of her mattress could cause excruciating pain. "How," she asked, "can I ever hold a job? How can I ever give back to the world that has given me so much?"

Morgan Amanda could not gird herself for yet another major surgery and yet another medical issue to contend with. She turned to her parents and requested palliative care. After twenty-six days in the hospital she moved to a hospice. It took two full weeks for the hospice team to get her pain under control, but she was finally at peace. A week later, Morgan Amanda died with her parents at her side, two weeks shy of her twenty-ninth birthday.

***

Shortly after completing this book, I was cleaning out a drawer full of papers. Among old IRS letters, crumpled but ever-optimistic to-do lists, and expired airline boarding passes, I came across a handwritten note on ivory card stock. The handwriting was tiny but neat, and filled every available space on the page. I scanned the text quickly—it was a thank-you note from someone I must have sent a copy of my earlier book to. The text ran flush against the bottom of the card so I couldn't read the scrawl of signature that was squeezed into the remaining nanometer of space. But it was a lovely letter, and I was touched by the author's kind words. I hunted for identifying information on the envelope but there was no name, only a street address in uncolored embossed letters. Elegant, I thought, but definitely not practical. Not enough contrast for me to read it, even *with* my reading glasses.

I examined the card again, and embossed on the front of the card—also in uncontrasted ivory letters—was an elegant monogram. I'd initially thought it was just an elaborately whorled design so didn't pay much attention, but now I could make out a sinuous F in the middle. And then I saw the smaller cursive M and A on either side of the F, the loops of all three joining in an old-fashioned calligraphic swirl.

MAF! It suddenly all fit together. I grabbed the envelope and squinted hard at the embossed address. Atlanta, Georgia—though it was honestly easier to feel than to read. I held the card under the brightest light I could find. Now that I knew what I was looking for, the minuscule scrawled signature had the topography of the words "Morgan Amanda."

I had completely forgotten about this letter! She had written it shortly after our meeting in New York, and I'd secured it in a drawer so as not to lose it, but it unfortunately got buried under a year's worth of paper sediment. I remembered being impressed that she'd written a formal thank-you both for our meeting and for the book I'd sent her some months earlier. I wasn't surprised, of course, by her attention to proper etiquette, but in an age awash with junk mail and spam, a handwritten note on monogrammed ivory stationery stands out.

"We can't have it all," she wrote to me in that card, "but we can try and succeed as long as we know and remember why we do it (and admit when we don't!)" That struck me as particularly emblematic of her approach to her life and to her illness. She also touched on the writing that she was working on and quoted Frida Kahlo: "I never painted dreams or nightmares. I paint my own reality." Then, so as not to take herself too seriously, she added a PS with an arrow that pointed to her elaborately looped monogram on the front. "PS: Isn't my MFA monogram hilarious? MFA—Master's in Fine Arts. Ha!" It was a standard-size thank-you card, but in many ways it personified Morgan Amanda. She had taken a small canvas and crammed it with as much life as she could. Every inch was filled with her humor, insights, generosity, and passion. Her life was not as long as it should have been, but she packed it to full capacity with everything she had.

CHAPTER 16

Can We Talk?

Evelyn Osorio is a fifty-six-year-old woman in my practice. Her diabetes and hypertension are relatively well-controlled but she's still twenty pounds heavier than she'd like to be. Her gym membership remains more theoretical than actual, though she now eats salad most days for lunch instead of pizza. She describes her life as stressful, though she's been good about keeping her appointments. She's someone who'd probably be described as a very average patient in a medical practice—a few mild-to-moderate illnesses, not excessively complicated from a medical perspective.

Nevertheless, my brain is racing during our visit. Even with a patient who is not especially ill there are dozens of thoughts scrambling in my head as we settle into our visit and begin talking.

- Blood sugar is a little better than last time. Have we checked her kidney function? Has she been to the eye doctor? The podiatrist?
- Cholesterol isn't ideal. Need to think about starting a statin, but she hates the idea of more meds.
- Darn, I forgot to return that phone call to Mr. Dayton. He's already left me three messages!
- Ms. Osorio's blood pressure is 148/93 today—okay but not great. Should we add another BP med? Will the greater number of pills risk less adherence?

- The computer is moving like oatmeal today. The traffic entering the Midtown Tunnel up the road is a veritable fleet of flitting gazelles by comparison. If I try to update the med list while I'm ordering labs the computer will probably flatline.
- Didn't Ms. Osorio mention last time that her husband was struggling at his job, maybe drinking a little more? Is she feeling just the regular stress of life, or might there be a clinical depression lurking underneath?
- Have we covered all of Ms. Osorio's health maintenance issues? When was her last mammogram? Has she had a colonoscopy since she turned fifty? Has she had a tetanus booster in the past ten years?
- These lousy keyboards inflame my carpal tunnel syndrome. If my right wrist conks out I'll never get through the next six patients. Plus my cello lesson is tomorrow. If I can't hold the bow properly I'll garble the Bach enough to cause all twenty of his offspring to yell for mercy from their graves.

Ms. Osorio interrupts my train of thought to tell me her back has been aching for the past few weeks. She's not interrupting, of course, she's just talking, but my brain has been bustling on overdrive so it feels like an interruption. From her perspective, this is the most important item in our visit, but unfortunately she's caught one of my neurons in midfire (the one that's thinking about her blood pressure, which is segueing into the neuron that's preparing the diet-and-exercise discussion, which is intersecting with the one that's debating whether the defibrillator on the crash cart might be an effective tool to goose up my crotchety computer).

My instinct is to put up one hand—the one without carpal tunnel—to keep all interruptions at bay till I've sorted everything out. It's not that I don't want to hear what she has to say, but the sensation that I'm juggling so many thoughts and need to resolve them all before the clock runs out keeps me in a moderate state of constant panic. What if I drop one? What if one of these critical thoughts evaporates while I address another concern and then I do something dangerous like prescribe a medication she's allergic to or miss an abnormal lab result?

I'm trying to type as fast as I can—for the very sake of not letting any thoughts escape—but every time I turn to the computer to write, I'm not making eye contact with Ms. Osorio. I know that eye contact is critically important for good communication and I don't want her to think the computer is more important than she is, but I have no choice but to keep looking toward the screen to dig out her blood tests, check the dates of her immunizations, type in the progress of her illnesses, order the labs for next time, refill her prescriptions, see what the gynecologist recommended.

Then she pulls out a form from her bag; her insurance company needs this form for some reason or another. An innocent—and completely justified—request, but this could be the straw that breaks the camel's back. The precarious balance of all that I'm keeping in the air could be unhinged by the appearance of an unassuming 8½-by-11-inch sheet of paper.

I try not to let my eyes widen with dismay, and indicate that we'll get to it after the physical exam. I barrel through the basics and quickly check for any red flag signs that might suggest her back pain is anything more than a routine muscle strain. I hustle back to the computer to input all the information, mentally running though my checklist, anxious that nothing important slip from my brain's increasingly tenuous holding bay.

I want to do everything properly and cover all our bases, but the more effort I place on accurate and thorough documentation, the less time I have to actually interact with my patient. A glance at the clock tells me we've gone well overtime. I struggle to wrap everything up, hoping I haven't forgotten anything important. I stand up and hand Mrs. Osorio her prescriptions, feeling more out of breath than an office visit should warrant.

"What about my insurance form?" she asks. "It needs to be in by Friday, otherwise I might lose my coverage."

I clap my hand against my forehead; I've completely forgotten about the form she'd asked about. It was hardly six minutes ago but my hippocampus evidently had hung out the next-cashier-please sign.

Numerous studies have debunked the myth of multitasking in humans. The concept of multitasking evolved from the computer field to explain a microprocessor performing two jobs at one time. It turns out that microprocessors are mostly linear and so are really performing only one task at a time. Computers give the *illusion* of simultaneous action by jumping between competing activities in a complex and rapid-paced algorithm.

Like microprocessors, we humans can't actually concentrate on two thoughts at the same exact time. We merely zip back and forth between them—with none of the algorithmic sophistication or breakneck speed of microprocessors—generally losing accuracy in the process. At most, we can juggle only a handful of thoughts in this desultory manner.

The more thoughts we juggle, the less we are able to attune fully to any given one. To me, this is a recipe for disaster. This time with Ms. Osorio I only forgot an insurance form. But what if I'd written the wrong dose on her prescription or refilled only five of her six medicines? What if I'd forgotten to fully explain the side effects of one of her meds? The list goes on, as does my fear of causing harm.

Interactions like this were one of the reasons I started writing this book. Ms. Osorio had several things she wanted to tell me, but I was hardly hearing them because of all the noise in my head. To be sure, most of that noise was about Ms. Osorio's medical care—with a few stray thoughts about phone messages, flitting gazelles, and the progeny of Bach—but I knew I wasn't fully attuned to what she was saying. At best, I could only keep half an ear on what she was saying, while my brain scurried around trying to stitch together the myriad elements of her medical care. And Ms. Osorio is a relatively uncomplicated patient; my sicker patients generate exponentially more balls in the air and the consequences of dropping any one are far graver.

The more researchers, patients, and doctors I spoke to for this book, the more I realized that our current setup in medicine seems designed to thwart good communication. There are so many odds stacked against it: a patient in pain or consumed with worry, a doctor with way too many tasks for the given time, uneven power dynamics, stereotypes, racial and gender disparities, assumptions, knowledge gaps. Add in ever more complex illnesses, exploding amounts of data for each patient, rigid documentation requirements, and ever-changing insurance company labyrinths to battle, and it's no wonder that a meaningful and well-understood conversation in the doctor's office is rarer than a decent cup of coffee from the hospital cafeteria.

The knowledge base and treatment options in medicine have exploded in the past half century of medicine, yet we still have the same fifteen-minute visit in which to accomplish everything. (And somehow, in this proliferative half century of scientific progress, we have never managed to improve upon the paper towel that passes for a gown.)

I know that my ideal world of luxurious hour-long visits will never come to pass. I'll never be able to fully barricade the exasperating bureaucracies, tyrannical telephones, and pseudo-time-saving technologies outside the door. (Though it sure is nice to fantasize . . .) But I remain convinced that it is possible to protect and even enhance doctor-patient communication, despite the multitude of factors conspiring against it.

Anatole Broyard observed, "Virginia Woolf [in her essay 'On Being Ill'] wondered why we don't have a greater literature of illness. The answer may be that doctors discourage our stories."[1] I've debated Broyard's harsh assessment and I'm not sure that doctors are as actively pernicious as he makes them out to be. I don't think doctors *intend* to discourage stories, but rather it is our system that makes full stories nearly impossible. By no means am I excusing doctors who don't at least make the effort, but I recognize that the problem is more than just doctors being paternalistic or wearing blinders.

The biggest take-home message for me, after wading through the research and interviewing people on all sides of the issue, is that both doctors and patients need to give communication its just due. Rather than seeing the conversation between doctor and patient as the utilitarian humdrum of a visit, the conversation should be viewed as the single most important tool of medical care. It should be given the deference and attention that we lavish upon the swankiest of medical technologies. If you consider the amount of information that can be gleaned from a doctor-patient conversation, the diagnoses that can be made, the analyses that can be elaborated, the treatments that can be rendered, the human connections that can be cultivated—the simple conversation is, in fact, a highly sophisticated technology. It's far more intricate, powerful, and flexible than most of our other medical technologies, which generally do only one thing in only one way. Plus, conversation is way cheaper and it doesn't decimate your sex drive or make you puke. (Except if you start talking about local politics . . .) The mere act of both parties taking this conversation more seriously will enhance communication and improve medical care. It's heartening to recognize that effective communication needn't take an unconscionably long time; it just needs full and intense focus. Such a focus, even for just a few minutes, can yield an abundance of information.

In his characteristic blunt yet philosophical style, Broyard put it this way: "I see no reason or need for my doctor to love me—nor would I expect him to suffer with me. I wouldn't demand a lot of my doctor's time: I just wish he would brood on my situation for perhaps five minutes, that he would give me his whole mind just once, be bonded with me for a brief space, survey my soul as well as my flesh, to get at my illness, for each man is ill in his own way."[2]

The giving of the whole mind is the key. For doctors, this means shunting aside competing thoughts, however virtuous and clinically relevant. I don't underestimate how onerous this task is, but doctors need to be fully focused on what the patient is saying because that's where nearly everything medically relevant resides.

The second thing doctors need to do is to shut up, at least a bit. The dogged detective instincts ingrained from medical training too often fly into overdrive, cutting off patients before they've hit their second syllable, racing down diagnostic pathways before the data have been fully collected. Misdiagnoses and medical errors flower in this wake. Holding back that first question bursting to erupt is agonizing for doctors; I feel your pain on this one. But if you can hold it for a minute, even thirty seconds, you'll be richly rewarded with better information, more accurate diagnoses, more efficient testing, improved adherence, and enhanced patient trust. And you'll probably even save time in the long run.

For the patient—who's often coming into the visit already feeling at a disadvantage—it's helpful to realize just how powerful the conversation is. In some ways, you hold all the cards; the story that you bring to your doctor is the essence of the medical visit. Insist that you be given time to tell your story. If your doctor jumps in too quickly, feel free to politely deflect. "Would it be okay if I had another minute to finish what I'm saying?" should do the trick.

If your doctor is excessively trigger happy with the questions, you could say something more direct like, "I need to finish telling you this. I'll keep it concise and as soon as I'm done, the floor is yours." And if she's completely tone deaf, you might have to look at her square in the face and say, "Listen, if you truly want to be efficient, just listen for two minutes so I can get my whole story out. *You'll* avoid diagnostic errors, and *I'll* avoid unnecessary tests."

Recognize, though, the reality of time and the limitations of how much can be accomplished in a single office visit. Invest some of your own time in advance preparation. Prioritize what you want to talk about and be realistic. If you press your doctors to address more than two or three issues in one visit, the focus and depth will necessarily be diluted. In fact, one of the things Corine Jansen now spends her time doing is helping patients—especially those with complicated illnesses—to develop an efficient, coherent narrative that clocks in at under three minutes. This allows both doctor and patient to focus fully on the main story, without competing distractions.

Before writing this book, I viewed communication little differently than I viewed breathing—both occurred automatically and I only really paid attention if they ceased. Communication wasn't on my to-do list for keeping up with medical advances. Whenever my periodic fits of medical spring cleaning occurred—those sporadic frenzies of self-improvement—I'd brush up on a couple of obscure physical exam skills, which of course I'd promptly never use in my daily practice. Or I'd spend a few weeks actually reading my medical journals rather than trying to osmose a smattering of facts by scanning the table of contents, feeling virtuous until the fever broke. But it never dawned on me to think critically and consciously about how I speak with my patients. I'd always thought I was a reasonably decent communicator (and frankly a pretty good breather as well).

When I turned the lens on my own practice, I observed that I fall short much more than I'd ever care to admit. I redirect the conversation within nanoseconds of the patient's chief complaint. My approach to improving adherence is always education and reeducation, reading the chronic-disease riot act at nearly every visit. Although my modus operandi is generally to be pleasant in conversational tone, there's no doubt I verbally dominate nearly every patient visit, shepherding the conversation along the most expeditious path possible. And I've never really stopped to think honestly about the biases that I bring into the exam room.

Each time I wrote about an experiment in this book, I tried to do a version of it in my own clinic sessions. It was about as effortless (and as comfortable) as resetting my breathing pattern to a polka rhythm. Every time was awkward and it often felt downright ridiculous. And I didn't necessarily see obvious results. I didn't suddenly turn into an orator extraordinaire, nor did my patients' blood pressures, glucose levels, and BMIs miraculously corral into glorious normalcy. But it turned out that the process, not the product, was the most valuable part.

My ingrained habits didn't rectify overnight but I did start noticing some of them. Usually it was only in retrospect, after the visit was over, that I recognized my blunders. But occasionally I could catch myself in the act. When my better angels were on duty I might actually be able to stop myself mid-harangue about becoming blind, impotent, amputated, and on dialysis (the monologue that my diabetic patients can no doubt recite from memory). It was no easy task to zip it up, for sure. But if I had my wits about me I could force the apocalypse faucet closed and simply ask, "What is the most challenging part of diabetes for you?" Nearly every time I had the presence of mind to switch gears like that, the patient came up with something specific, rather than the abstract horrors I was honking on about ad nauseam. I could then note down that challenge in the chart, and we'd have something real to focus on. And beyond providing a more practical direction for our medical efforts, the exchange offered me singular insights into this individual's life with diabetes. Disease is never abstract for a patient, and it's only by foraying into the particulars that a doctor can ever begin to fathom the unique trek of illness that each patient must navigate.

When I'm not too overwhelmed with the logistical tribulations of the day, I try to experiment with some of the other techniques I read about: asking a patient to "share back" what we've just discussed, adding in an extra dose of optimism about a treatment, matching my medical terminology to my patient's, stepping back from my natural tendency to steer the visit in the way my inner racehorse deems most time-efficient. They don't all work all the time, and there's no magic, but stirring the pot in a variety of ways almost always brings something of import to our medical encounter. And if nothing else, the conversation is far more interesting for both of us.

The hardest thing by far is trying to rout out my biases. No doubt they are so ingrained culturally and personally that I'm not even aware of most of them. But I'm making an effort to notice them, and to confront them when I find them. When I read a patient's name on the chart, for example, I try to pay attention as to whether my mind is racing ahead with predictions and assumptions before I've actually met the person. I can't always stop these snap judgments, but I *can* administer a mental kick in the shins if needed. I'm also trying to consider more explicitly which biases my patients may have faced in prior medical experiences and how these might impact my encounter with them. Some of my patients have suffered concrete offenses at the hands of the medical system, and the resulting wariness is often interpreted as "noncompliance." I can't undo all the societal injustices out there but I *can* think carefully about whether I'm promulgating them.

Thankfully, we seem to be evolving from the old-school view that considered communication merely an affable bonus that a few kindly doctors possess. You'll still occasionally hear that so-and-so is an excellent doctor even though he has a bedside manner that rivals a roll of surgical tape. But increasingly we are recognizing that this is a contradiction: you can't *be* an excellent doctor if you have a lousy bedside manner. Communication is not an extraneous perk but rather the bedrock of high-quality medical care. Without good communication between doctors and patients, the chances of achieving effective medical outcomes plummet.

Human connection is a seedling that needs to be cultivated, and good communication is the loam in which it is nurtured. The doctor-patient relationship is a particular human connection, one that carries uniquely high stakes—health and even life can hang in the balance. Communication between doctor and patient, therefore, assumes these stakes.

If well tended with appropriate respect, attention, and time, this communication will take root, nourishing a sturdy doctor-patient relationship. What can be reaped—easing of suffering, improvement of health, solidification of connection—helps enhance our lives on both sides of the stethoscope.

When I think back to my communicative mishaps with Oumar Amadou, my patient from the opening of the book, I can see more clearly how and why it was so exasperating. The geometry of our conversation went awry as we pursued divergent dialogues. Although I appreciated the severity of his cardiac disease, I was irritated by the muscularity of his insistence and quickly pegged him as a "difficult patient." In retrospect, I can see that my labeling of him created a bias that distorted what I heard. In his persistent demands for my time, I discerned entitlement. I became resentful and grew impatient with him.

Had I stopped talking for a bit, stopped arguing about appointments and phone calls, I might have been able to intuit the animating impulse of his desperation. Mr. Amadou was wrestling with the very real demons that his heart disease dealt out and he was in a justified existential panic.

Those of us whose luck has kept us from facing down death can't really appreciate the exquisite vulnerability that serious disease engenders. Raw fear is a motivating force like no other. When I try to imagine what it would feel like to be Mr. Amadou—navigating a complex and unforgiving medical system, negotiating in an unfamiliar language, all with a heart that had proved itself unreliable long before its warranty was up—I can begin to understand his approach. Why *wouldn't* he—like Morgan Amanda—insist on what he perceived as necessary? Why *wouldn't* he refuse to take no for an answer? But I wasn't able to fully comprehend that until his body crumpled in my office and I felt the life wicking away from him.

After his faulty pacemaker was replaced and the excess fluid drained from his lungs, Mr. Amadou came for a post-discharge appointment. It was an almost intolerable relief to see his lanky frame in his trusty tracksuit filling my doorway. When I shook his hand—the hand that had been chillingly frigid the last time I'd held it—I basked in its ardent warmth. I had no illusions, of course, and neither did he. The recent tune-up did not impart any fairy dust of additional cardiac reserve. Mr. Amadou would not be doing the two-hundred-meter dash down Lexington Avenue anytime soon.

But we'd dodged the bullet, this time at least, and we both exhaled cautious sighs of relief. Mr. Amadou's first question, of course, was when our next appointment would be. Normally, this would irritate me, but now his voice unfurled almost like a benediction, so relieved was I that he had survived.

I couldn't promise that we'd never have any miscommunications in the future, or that I—or he—wouldn't get aggravated when things didn't work out as swimmingly as we'd like. But I *could* promise that I would pay more attention to how I listened and how I spoke. I couldn't realign his obstreperous cardiac myocytes, but I could commit to more conscientious communication.

When poet John Stone offered the graduating medical students his indelible commencement poem, he told them: "You will learn to see most acutely out of the corner of your eye, to hear best with your inner ear."[3] A more astute lesson in communication I could hardly imagine.

Acknowledgments

The idea of this book arose from conversations with Morgan Amanda Fritzlen and Juliet Mavromatis. I want to thank them for their generosity of time, experience, and spirit. Morgan Amanda, you are very much missed.

Much appreciation to David Baron, Tracey Pratt, Marije Klein, Corine Jansen, and Debra Roter who spent hours sharing their stories with me, and answering dozens of follow-up e-mails. Thank you also to Jerrice and Tom Fritzlen, Heidi E. Hamilton, Annie Brewster, Ted Kaptchuk, Eric Simon, Richard Street, Graham Bodie, Janet Bavelas, Steve Kraman, Carol Liebman, Roel Straathof, Jane Ogden, Donald Boudreau, and Peter Lewy. There are also many others who kindly shared their thoughts, but there simply wasn't room in the book for all of these incredible stories.

I am extremely grateful to my patients, who've taught me so much about medicine and about being a doctor. A special thanks to my colleagues at Bellevue and NYU who have been so supportive over the years. Some anecdotes in this book previously appeared in the *New York Times* and the *Los Angeles Times*. Thank you to those editors, especially to Toby Bilanow of the *New York Times*, for helping to shape and give life to those stories.

An enormous and ongoing thanks to Helene Atwan—my editor and publisher—for showing nothing but optimism, enthusiasm, and astute editorial eyes all along the way. Gratitude to Pam MacColl, Tom Hallock, Alyssa Hassan, and the entire team at Beacon Press for their meticulous work and endless encouragement. In the publishing world where editorial teams are typically upended more frequently than the spin cycle on a dryer, to have worked with Helene,

Pam, and Tom through five books over fifteen years might qualify for a Guinness world record, or at the very least a round of Guinness stout.

My children—Naava, Noah, and Ariel—quip that each of their entrances into the family was timed to a book. It wasn't quite planned that way, but fifteen years ago, in the acknowledgments for my first book, I thanked Naava for teaching me the fine art of editing on a computer while nursing. Now I can thank the crew (and I'd be pilloried if I left out our trusty Lab-mutt, Juliet) for teaching me the more formidable but more fun art of concentrating amid chaos. It's boisterous but never boring, amply stocked with whole-wheat-everything bagels, dog biscuits, cutthroat backgammon, and musical grit.

My everlasting gratitude is to my husband, Benjy Akman—trouper extraordinaire—who has survived these books and all the associated tumult and travel with peerless aplomb. No matter who was in crisis over a science fair project, or whose violin string had popped, or how little milk was left in the fridge or how much barking there was in the background, he'd always take care of it all with a smile and say, "Everything's fine. Go enjoy!" It's been quite the lively book we've shared thus far, and I can't wait to see what the next chapter brings.

Notes

CHAPTER 1: COMMUNICATION AND ITS DISCONTENTS

1. Pseudonym. The names of the patients in this book have been changed to protect their identities, with the exception of Morgan Amanda Fritzlen and Tracey Pratt, who consented to have their real names used. Non-patient names are real.

CHAPTER 2: FROM BOTH SIDES NOW

1. H. T. Tu and J. R. Lauer, "Word of Mouth and Physician Referrals Still Drive Health Care Provider Choice," *Research Briefs* 9 (2008): 1–8.

2. Research of Kahneman and Tversky summarized in Daniel Kahneman, *Thinking Fast and Slow* (New York: Farrar, Straus and Giroux, 2011).

3. A. Victoor et al., "Determinants of Patient Choice of Healthcare Providers: A Scoping Review," *BMC Health Services Research* 12 (2012): 272–88; K. M. Harris et al., "How Do Patients Choose Physicians? Evidence from a National Survey of Enrollees in Employment-Related Health Plans," *Health Services Research* 38 (2003): 711–32.

4. M. Wensing et al., "A Systematic Review of the Literature on Patient Priorities for General Practice Care, Part 1: Description of the Research," *Social Science & Medicine* 47 (1998): 1573–88; A. Coulter, "What Do Patients and the Public Want from Primary Care?" *British Medical Journal* 331 (2005): 1199–1201.

5. D. R. Rhoades et al., "Speaking and Interruptions During Primary Care Office Visits," *Family Medicine* 33 (2001): 528–32.

CHAPTER 3: IT TAKES TWO

1. S. Morgan, "Miscommunication Between Patients and General Practitioners: Implications for Clinical Practice," *Journal of Primary Health Care* 5 (2013): 123–28.

2. M. Marvel et al., "Soliciting the Patient's Agenda: Have We Improved?" *Journal of the American Medical Association* 281 (1999): 283–87.

3. W. Langewitz et al., "Spontaneous Talking Time at Start of Consultation in Outpatient Clinic: Cohort Study," *British Medical Journal* 325 (2002): 682–83.

CHAPTER 4: NOW HEAR THIS

1. Josh Mitchell, "Women Notch Progress," *Wall Street Journal*, December 4, 2012.

2. On the rate of doctors who are women, see "Distribution of Physicians by Gender," State Health Facts, Henry J. Kaiser Family Foundation, April 2016. On the rate of medical students who are women, see "Table A-7, Applicants, First-Time Applicants, Acceptees, and Matriculants to U.S. Medical Schools by Sex, 2006-2007 Through 2015-2016," Association of American Medical Colleges.

3. J. A. Hall, D. L. Roter, and C. S. Rand, "Communication of Affect Between Patient and Physician," *Journal of Health and Social Behavior* 22 (1981): 18–30.

4. D. L. Roter, "Patient Participation in the Patient-Provider Interaction: The Effects of Patient Question Asking on the Quality of Interaction, Satisfaction and Compliance," *Health Education & Behavior* 5 (1977): 281–315.

5. T. S. Inui et al., "Outcome-Based Doctor-Patient Interaction Analysis: I. Comparison of Techniques," *Medical Care* 20 (1982): 535–49.

6. D. L. Roter et al., "Communication Patterns of Primary Care Physicians," *Journal of the American Medical Association* 277 (1997): 350–56.

CHAPTER 5: WITH ALL GOOD INTENTIONS

1. H. E. Hamilton, "Patients' Voices in the Medical World: An Exploration of Accounts of Noncompliance," in *Georgetown University Roundtable on Languages and Linguistics*, ed. D. Tannen and J. E. Alatis (Washington, DC: Georgetown University Press, 2001), 147–65.

2. M. T. Brown and J. K. Bussell, "Medication Adherence: Who Cares?," *Mayo Clinic Proceedings* 86 (2011): 304–14.

3. A. Schoenthaler et al., "Patient-Physician Communication Is an Important Predictor of Medication Adherence in Hypertensive Patients" (paper under review).

4. P. ten Have, "Talk and Institution: A Reconsideration of the 'Asymmetry' of Doctor-Patient Interaction," in *Talk and Social Structure*, ed. Deirdre Boden and Don H. Zimmerman (Berkeley: University of California Press, 1991), 138–63.

5. A. Brewster, "Storytelling for Health: Doctor Promotes Intimate Patient Narratives," *CommonHealth*, WBUR, March 11, 2014.

6. A. Brewster and J. Adler, "Boundary Crossing: When Doctors and Patients Get Personal for Better Health," *CommonHealth*, WBUR, January 1, 2015.

7. Ibid.

CHAPTER 6: WHAT WORKS

1. L. D. Egbert et al., "Reduction of Postoperative Pain by Encouragement and Instruction of Patients—A Study of Doctor-Patient Rapport," *New England Journal of Medicine* 270 (1964): 825–87.

2. International Federation of Health Plans, *2013 Comparative Price Report: Variation in Medical and Hospital Prices by Country*, 2013 (accessed June 17, 2016).

3. J. Fuentes et al., "Enhanced Therapeutic Alliance Modulates Pain Intensity and Muscle Pain Sensitivity in Patients with Chronic Low Back Pain: An Experimental Controlled Study," *Physical Therapy* 94 (2014) 477–89.

4. M. Amanzio et al., "Response Variability to Analgesics: A Role for Nonspecific Activation of Endogenous Opioids," *Pain* 90 (2001): 205–15.

5. J. D. Levine et al., "The Mechanism of Placebo Analgesia," *Lancet* 8091 (1978): 654–57.

6. A. Goldstein et al., "A Synthetic Peptide with Morphine-like Pharmacologic Action," *Life Sciences* 17 (1975): 1643–54.

7. T. J. Kaptchuk et al., "Placebos Without Deception: A Randomized Controlled Trial in Irritable Bowel Syndrome," *PLoS ONE* 12 (2010): e15591.

8. S. C. Hull et al., "Patients' Attitudes About the Use of Placebo Treatments: Telephone Survey," *British Medical Journal* 347 (2013): f3757.

9. U. Bingel et al., "The Effect of Treatment Expectation on Drug Efficacy: Imaging the Analgesic Benefit of the Opioid Remifentanil," *Science Translational Medicine* 3 (2011).

10. M. R. DiMatteo, "Variations in Patients' Adherence to Medical Recommendations: A Quantitative Review of 50 Years of Research," *Medical Care* 42 (2004): 200–209.

11. K. B. Haskard Zolnierek and M. R. Dimatteo, "Physician Communication and Patient Adherence to Treatment: A Meta-Analysis," *Medical Care* 47 (2009) 826–34.

12. S. H. McDaniel et al., "Physician Self-Disclosure in Primary Care Visits: Enough About You, What About Me?," *Archives of Internal Medicine* 167 (2007): 1321–26.

13. D. S. Morse et al., "Enough About Me, Let's Get Back to You: Physician Self-Disclosure During Primary Care Encounters," *Annals of Internal Medicine* 149, no. 11 (2008): 835–37.

14. M. C. Beach et al., "Is Physician Self-Disclosure Related to Patient Evaluation of Office Visits?," *Journal of General Internal Medicine* 19 (2004): 905–10.

15. M. Hojat et al., "Physician Empathy: Definition, Measurement, and Relationship to Gender and Specialty," *American Journal of Psychiatry* 159 (2002): 1563–69.

16. M. Hojat et al., Physicians' Empathy and Clinical Outcomes for Diabetic Patients," *Academic Medicine* 86 (2011): 359–64.

17. D. Rakel et al., "Perception of Empathy in the Therapeutic Encounter: Effects on the Common Cold," *Patient Education and Counseling* 85 (2011): 390–97.

18. R. L. Street Jr. et al., "How Does Communication Heal? Pathways Linking Clinician-Patient Communication to Health Outcomes," *Patient Education and Counseling* 74 (2009): 295–301.

19. J. K Rao et al., "Communication Interventions Make a Difference in Conversations Between Physicians and Patients: A Systematic Review of the Evidence," *Medical Care* 45 (2007): 340–49.

CHAPTER 8: LISTEN TO ME

1. J. B. Bavelas et al., "Listeners as Co-Narrators," *Journal of Personality and Social Psychology* 79 (2000): 941–52.

2. H. Korman et al., "Microanalysis of Formulations in Solution-Focused Brief Therapy, Cognitive Behavioral Therapy, and Motivational Interviewing," *Journal of Systemic Therapies* 32 (2013): 32–46.

3. H. H. Clark and S. A. Brennan, "Grounding in Communication," in *Perspectives on Socially Shared Cognition*, ed. L. B. Resnick, J. M. Levine, and S. D. Teasley (Washington, DC: APA Books, 1991).

4. J. B. Bavelas et al., "Beyond Back-Channels: A Three-Step Model of Grounding in Face-to-Face Dialogue," abstract presented at the Interdisciplinary Workshop on Feedback Behaviors in Dialog, Stevenson, WA, September 2012.

CHAPTER 9: JUST THE FACTS, MA'AM

1. A. N. Makaryus and E. A. Friedman, "Patients' Understanding of Their Treatment Plans and Diagnosis at Discharge," *Mayo Clinic Proceedings* 80 (2005) 991–94.

2. D. P. Olson and D. M. Windish, "Communication Discrepancies Between Physicians and Hospitalized Patients," *Archives of Internal Medicine* 170 (2010): 1302–7.

3. K. J. O'Leary et al., "Hospitalized Patients' Understanding of Their Plan of Care," *Mayo Clinic Proceedings* 85 (2010): 47–52.

4. R. P. C. Kessels, "Patients' Memory for Medical Information," *Journal of the Royal Society of Medicine* 96 (2003) 219–22.

5. J. S. Albrecht et al., "Hospital Discharge Instructions: Comprehension and Compliance Among Older Adults," *Journal of General Internal Medicine* 11 (2012): 1491–98; L. I. Horwitz et al., "Quality of Discharge Practices and Patient Understanding at an Academic Medical Center," *JAMA Internal Medicine* 173 (2013): 1715–22; K. W. Heng et al., "Recall of Discharge Advice Given to Patients with Minor Head Injury Presenting to a Singapore Emergency Department," *Singapore Medical Journal* 12 (2007): 1107–10.

6. J. Silberman et al., "Recall-Promoting Physician Behaviors in Primary Care," *Journal of General Internal Medicine* 23 (2008): 1487–90.

7. S. Kripalani et al., "Clinical Research in Low-Literacy Populations: Using Teach-Back to Assess Comprehension of Informed Consent and Privacy Information," *IRB* 30 (2008): 13–9; C. Teutsch, "Patient-Doctor Communication," *Medical Clinics of North America* 87 (2003): 1115–45.

8. C. F. Kellett et al., "Poor Recall Performance of Journal-Browsing Doctors," *Lancet* 348 (1996): 479.

9. V. L. Patel, "Differences Between Medical Students and Doctors in Memory for Clinical Cases," *Medical Education* 20 (1986): 3–9.

10. J. L. Coulehan et al., "'Let Me See If I Have This Right . . .': Words That Help Build Empathy," *Annals of Internal Medicine* 135 (2001): 221–27.

CHAPTER 10: DO NO HARM

1. H. B. Beckman et al., "The Doctor-Patient Relationship and Malpractice: Lessons from Plaintiff Depositions," *Archives of Internal Medicine* 154 (1994): 1365–70.

2. R. S. Shapiro et al., "A Survey of Sued and Nonsued Physicians and Suing Patients," *Archives of Internal Medicine* 149 (1989): 2190–96.

3. W. Levinson et al., "Physician-Patient Communication: The Relationship with Malpractice Claims Among Primary Care Physicians and Surgeons," *Journal of the American Medical Association* 277 (1997): 553–59.

4. N. Ambady et al., "Surgeons' Tone of Voice: A Clue to Malpractice History," *Surgery* 132 (2002): 5–9.

5. C. B. Liebman and C. S. Hyman, "A Mediation Skills Model to Manage Disclosure of Errors and Adverse Events to Patients," *Health Affairs* 23 (2004): 22–32.

6. S. S. Kraman and G. Hamm, "Risk Management: Extreme Honesty May Be the Best Policy," *Annals of Internal Medicine* 131 (1999): 963–67.

7. A. Kachalia et al., "Liability Claims and Costs Before and After Implementation of a Medical Error Disclosure Program," *Annals of Internal Medicine* 153 (2010): 213–21.

8. JoNel Aleccia, "Nurse's Suicide Highlights Twin Tragedies of Medical Errors," NBCNews.com, June 27, 2010.

9. T. H. Gallagher et al., "Patients' and Physicians' Attitudes Regarding the Disclosure of Medical Errors," *Journal of the American Medical Association* 289 (2003): 1001–7.

10. A. W. Wu et al., "Disclosing Medical Errors to Patients: It's Not What You Say, It's What They Hear," *Journal of General Internal Medicine* 24, no. 9 (2009): 1012–17.

CHAPTER 11: WHAT LIES BENEATH

1. Wendell Berry, "Health Is Membership," in *Another Turn of the Crank* (Berkeley, CA: Counterpoint Press, 1995).

2. M. Peltenburg et al., "The Unexpected in Primary Care: A Multicenter Study on the Emergence of Unvoiced Patient Agenda," *Annals of Family Medicine* 2 (2004): 534–40.

3. J. White et al., "'Oh, by the Way': The Closing Moments of the Medical Visit," *Journal of General Internal Medicine* 9 (1994): 24–28.

4. S. Sprague et al., "Prevalence of Intimate Partner Violence Across Medical and Surgical Health Care Settings," *Violence Against Women* 20 (2014): 118–36.

5. A. A. Guth and L. Pachter, "Domestic Violence and the Trauma Surgeon," *American Journal of Surgery* 179 (2000): 134–40.

6. National Assessment of Adult Literacy, 2003 survey, National Center for Education Statistics, Institute of Education Sciences.

7. "Health Literacy," National Network of Libraries of Medicine, 2013.

8. S. Kripalani et al., "Health Literacy and the Quality of Physician-Patient Communication During Hospitalization," *Journal of Hospital Medicine* 5 (2010): 269–75; N. D. Berkman et al., "Low Health Literacy and Health Outcomes: An Updated Systematic Review," *Annals of Internal Medicine* 155 (2011): 97–107.

CHAPTER 12: THE LANGUAGE OF MEDICINE

1. A. Tailor and J. Ogden, "Avoiding the Term 'Obesity': An Experimental Study of the Impact of Doctors' Language on Patients' Beliefs," *Patient Education and Counseling* 76 (2009): 260–64.

2. M. Tayler and J. Ogden, "Doctors' Use of Euphemisms and Their Impact on Patients' Beliefs About Health: An Experimental Study of Heart Failure," *Patient Education and Counseling* 57 (2005).

3. N. Williams and J. Ogden, "The Impact of Matching the Patient's Vocabulary: A Randomized Control Trial," *Family Practice* 21 (2004): 630–35.

4. J. Ogden, and K. Parkes, "'A Diabetic' Versus 'A Person with Diabetes': The Impact of Language on Beliefs about Diabetes," *European Diabetes Nursing* 10 (2013): 80–85.

5. P. Burdett-Smith, "On the Naming of the Parts," *British Medical Journal* 311 (1995): 1406.

6. J. Blackman and M. Sahebjalal, "Patient Understanding of Frequently Used Cardiology Terminology," *British Journal of Cardiology* 29 (2014): 39.

7. From John Stone, *Renaming the Streets* (Baton Rouge: Louisiana State University Press, 1985).

CHAPTER 13: RUSHING TO JUDGMENT?

1. M. M. Huizinga et al., "Physician Respect for Patients with Obesity," *Journal of General Internal Medicine* 24 (2009): 1236–39.

2. K. A. Gudzune et al., "Physicians Build Less Rapport with Obese Patients," *Obesity* 21 (2013): 2146–52.

3. R. M. Puhl et al., "The Effect of Physicians' Body Weight on Patient Attitudes: Implications for Physician Selection, Trust and Adherence to Medical Advice," *International Journal of Obesity* 37 (2013): 1415–21.

4. B. D. Smedley, A. Y. Stith, and A. R. Nelson, eds., *Unequal Treatment: Confronting Racial and Ethnic Disparities in Healthcare* (Washington, DC: National Academies Press, 2003).

5. R. L. Johnson et al., "Patient Race/Ethnicity and Quality of Patient-Physician Communication During Medical Visits," *American Journal of Public Health* 94 (2004): 2084–90.

6. L. A. Cooper et al., "Patient-Centered Communication, Ratings of Care, and Concordance of Patient and Physician Race," *Annals of Internal Medicine* 139 (2003): 907–15.

7. A. G. Greenwald et al., "Measuring Individual Differences in Implicit Cognition: The Implicit Association Test," *Journal of Personality and Social Psychology* 74 (1988): 1464–80.

8. L. A. Cooper et al., "The Associations of Clinicians' Implicit Attitudes About Race with Medical Visit Communication and Patient Ratings of Interpersonal Care," *American Journal of Public Health* 102 (2012): 979–87.

9. I. V. Blair et al., "Clinicians' Implicit Ethnic/Racial Bias and Perceptions of Care Among Black and Latino Patients," *Annals of Family Medicine* 11 (2013): 43–52.

10. J. A. Sabin et al., "Physicians' Implicit and Explicit Attitudes About Race by MD Race, Ethnicity, and Gender," *Journal of Health Care for the Poor and Underserved* 20 (2009): 896–913.

11. L. R. M. Hausmann et al., "Impact of Perceived Discrimination in Health Care on Patient-Provider Communication," *Medical Care* 49 (2011): 626–33.

12. K. D. Martin et al., "Physician Communication Behaviors and Trust Among Black and White Patients with Hypertension," *Medical Care* 51 (2013): 151–57.

13. B. B. Drwecki et al., "Reducing Racial Disparities in Pain Treatment: The Role of Empathy and Perspective-Taking," *Pain* 152 (2011): 1001–6.

14. V. W. Chang et al., "Quality of Care Among Obese Patients," *Journal of the American Medical Association* 303 (2010): 1274–81.

CHAPTER 14: CAN IT BE TAUGHT?

1. J. D. Boudreau et al., "Preparing Medical Students to Become Attentive Listeners," *Medical Teacher* 31 (2009): 22–29.

2. L. Fallowfield et al., "Enduring Impact of Communication Skills Training: Results of a 12-Month Follow-up," *British Journal of Cancer* 8 (2003): 1445–49.

3. C. A. Lee et al., "Standardized Patient-Narrated Web-Based Learning Modules Improve Students' Communication Skills on a High-Stakes Clinical Skills Examination," *Journal of General Internal Medicine* 26 (2011): 1374–77.

4. D. L. Roter et al., "The Impact of Patient and Physician Computer Mediated Communication Skill Training on Reported Communication and Patient Satisfaction," *Patient Education and Counseling* 88 (2012): 406–13.

5. J. K. Rao et al., "Communication Interventions Make a Difference in Conversations Between Physicians and Patients: A Systematic Review of the Evidence," *Medical Care* 45 (2007): 340–49.

6. Anatole Broyard, *Intoxicated by My Illness: And Other Writings on Life and Death* (New York: Fawcett Columbine, 1992), 43.

7. D. E. Epner et al., "Difficult Conversations: Teaching Medical Oncology Trainees Communication Skills One Hour at a Time," *Academic Medicine* 89 (2014): 578–84.

CHAPTER 16: CAN WE TALK?

1. Broyard, *Intoxicated by My Illness*, 52.

2. Ibid., 44.

3. From "Gaudeamus Igitur" in Stone, *Renaming the Streets*.

Index